SHIATSU

Japanese Finger

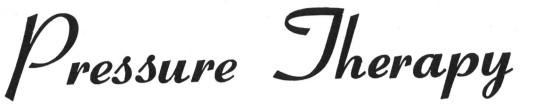

Pressure Therapy

SHIATSU

by **Tokujiro Namikoshi**

JAPAN PUBLICATIONS, INC. Publishers

THIS IS A POPULAR VERSION OF *SHIATSU: HEALTH AND VITALITY AT YOUR FINGERTIPS* BY THE SAME AUTHOR AND PUBLISHERS.

Published by JAPAN PUBLICATIONS, INC. Distributed by JAPAN PUBLICATIONS TRADING COMPANY, 1255 Howard St., San Francisco, Calif. 94103; P.O. Box 5030, Tokyo International, Tokyo, Japan. © 1969 by JAPAN PUBLICATIONS, INC. Printed in Japan by Ichimura Color Photo. Printing Co., Ltd.   Layout and Typography by Soshichi Toyoshima

Library of Congress Catalog Card No. 68–19983
ISBN 0–87040–169–6

First Edition, 1972
Second Printing: October, 1972
Third Printing: April, 1973
Fourth Printing: September, 1973

Preface

SHIATSU, the finger-pressure therapy, can give new stamina to the office worker and can spur him on to achievements he never dreamed possible. The teacher who tries it will find himself able to turn dullards into top-grade scholars; the wife who knows shiatsu will have a more contented, healthier husband. If you try it on your own body you will soon both look better and feel better. Shiatsu can help you guard against colds, stomach disorders, cerebral hemorrhage, and even cancer. Some of you may think that in claiming such results I am going too far, but, at the risk of sounding boastful, I would like to say that I have been a specialist in this field for forty-two years and that I have given satisfaction to more than 100,000 patients. I am the founder of the Nippon Shiatsu School, now in its twenty-eight years, which has graduated 20,000 qualified shiatsu specialists. I have written this book, as the product of my many years of experience, in the firm belief that shiatsu can help each individual to a healthier, more constructive life. Since I feel that, in our age, we must offer what we know to others in the hope of building a better society now, in my early sixties, I have poured into this work the essence of all my knowledge. This book represents the heart of shiatsu treatment.

Whereas in some cases a short shiatsu period is adequate, other cases require longer. My basic aim is to convince the people of today, already prone to rely too heavily on medicines and shots, that even brief shiatsu treatments can reveal the truly astounding life powers of the human body.

TOKUJIRO NAMIKOSHI

Contents

Preface
Contents
Cautions about the Use of Shiatsu

Chapter Four: SHIATSU TREATMENT FOR SPECIFIC
                ILLNESSES

Cautions about the Use of Shiatsu

This book is intended to help the average person ease slight daily pains and aches and to promote health and well-being in the entire body. Reading it does not give anyone sufficient knowledge to apply the shiatsu method to seriously ill patients. I myself, after long years of shiatsu experience, always consult a physician before beginning treatment on difficult cases. To apply thorough shiatsu, one must completely understand the body of the patient.

To avoid possible trouble, I suggest that the reader heed the following cautionary remarks.

1. Do not attempt treatment of contagious diseases: osteomyelitis, influenza, hydrophobia, jaundice, contagious diarrhea, whooping cough, measles, yellow fever, malaria, Japanese river fever, filaria, tropical fever.

2. **Do not treat patients with a series of internal disorders** of the heart, liver, kidneys or lungs.

3. Do not treat patients susceptible to internal bleeding from external stimuli: cases of purpura, haemophilia, stomach ulcers, duodenal ulcers, aneurism.

4. Do not treat patients with cancer of the stomach, intestine or uterus, or those with sarcoma.

5. Do not treat patients who have just fractured a bone or who have a twisted intestine.

6. Remember, though serious illness responds to shiatsu, ONLY AN EXPERIENCED SHIATSU SPECIALIST SHOULD TREAT THEM.

CHAPTER ONE

Introduction

Shiatsu

The word "shiatsu," composed of the elements *shi* (fingers) and *atsu* (pressure), means a method of treating illness with digital compression. The basis of the science is pure instinct. After all, a person tired from too much golf or television, or from typing for long hours at a stretch instinctively rubs or massages the part of the body that hurts or feels cramped and stiff. Over the past forty years of study of human movement and research in therapy, I have evolved the system of shiatsu, which not only cures illness, but also promotes greater stamina and mental composure and can even help married couples lead a happier matrimonial life. Having treated over 100,000 patients and seen more than 20,000 students graduate from the Nippon Shiatsu School, I always insist that

"The heart of shiatsu is like pure maternal affection;
The pressure of the hands causes the springs of life to flow."

Manual Therapy

In most manual therapy methods, whether Occidental massage or Japanese *amma,* the effect, usually no more than recovery of movement in some part of the body, is more superficial than the deep treatment achieved by shiatsu compression, perpendicularly applied with the balls of the thumbs. Widely practiced in Japan today, shiatsu is described by the Ministry of Welfare as follows:

Shiatsu is a treatment in which the thumbs and palms of the hands are used to apply pressure to certain points in order to correct irregularities of the living body, maintain or improve health, and contribute to the cure of certain illnesses.

Making Use of the Body's Own Power

Not merely a remedy, shiatsu, relying on the mental attitude of the person undergoing treatment, stimulates the generation of power to prevent illness.

In 1953, a group of chiropractic schools invited me to lecture in various parts of the United States. In Los Angeles, during one of a three-day series of talks, a watchmaker in the audience asked me the following question.

"I am a watchmaker. It takes me three years to train a watch repairman. How can you explain in only three days how to repair the human body, which is much more complex than a watch?"

I replied that his question was reasonable but that he should remember two things: first, a watch is only a machine; second, the human body has powers of regeneration and self-repair which no machine can equal. For instance, when a foreign object falls into the eye, tears immediately wash it away; when a bite of food or a little liquid goes into the trachea, the person naturally coughs to dislodge it. Scraped skin grows back in a few days. In other words, the body can do so much of its own repair that we need no repairmen.

I went on to say that shiatsu can work apparent miracles because it uses the natural instinct to press ailing parts of the body and because it takes advantage of the body's wonderful natural powers. Certainly, some few scientific points need explanation, but the real purpose of my talks is simply to have you realize the power inherent in the body and use it by applying pressure where it is needed. The watchmaker seemed convinced.

Depending too much on doctors, drugs, and injections, people today tend to overlook the importance of natural cure. Hippocrates, the father of medicine, had just such cure in mind when he said that nature is medicine and medicine the servant of nature. The people who coined the proverb, "Nature cures the illness, but the doctor gets the fee," were thinking along the same lines.

All the tense, nervous semi-invalids crowding doctors offices would be much better off if they opened their eyes to the miracles the body can do by itself. Shiatsu tries to help open some of those eyes.

The Effect of Shiatsu

About 450 muscles, attached to bones at either end, by contracting, produce movement in the human body. The contraction results from a complex process beginning when nutrients from food digested in the stomach are absorbed through the duodenum and pass to the liver, where they are converted into glycogen. Distributed through the blood stream to the muscles, glycogen combines with oxygen from the lungs and by combustion generates energy for muscular contraction. The process produces a residue, called lactic acid, which causes the fatigue element. That is, when sufficient lactic acid accumulates in the muscle, contraction becomes either difficult or impossible.

Exhaustion, caused by an over-accumulation of lactic acid in the muscles, can be relieved by suspending muscular contraction for a while, in other words, by taking a rest. As the lactic acid is carried away in the veins, new glycogen is brought in by the arteries to provide a fresh source of energy for muscular action. If the fatigue element goes uncorrected for a long time, the muscles contract improperly, thus producing irregularities in the skeleton and disturbances in the blood vessels, nerves, and lymph ducts in the muscles. The result is illness.

By applying digital pressure over a muscle that contracts improperly because of an over-accumulation of lactic acid, it is possible to cause 80 per cent of that acid to reconvert into glycogen. This eliminates fatigue and, with it, improper muscular contraction, the cause of illness.

Shiatsu Is Open to Everyone

Although complicated illnesses require the attention of shiatsu specialists, with a basic knowledge of the anatomy of the human body (Fig. 5 and 54) and with the foundation in shiatsu techniques offered in this book, anyone can perform simple treatments that will relieve fatigue, aching shoulders, backaches, toothaches, high blood pressure, and even bedwetting. Not only is it possible to use shiatsu to make life more comfortable and healthful for others, it is also beneficial to apply the techniques to oneself. For instance, I give myself a good shiatsu treatment each time I take a bath, and I find that I feel much better for it.

Using the Fingers

Active manual participation in shiatsu optimizes the treatment's effect by stimulating the circulation of the blood to the fingertips and preventing blood congestion in other parts of the body. The source of the body's nourishment, blood, naturally flows to the areas in use at the moment: when one eats it flows to the stomach, and when one thinks, it flows to the brain. Since the nerves in the fingertips are directly connected with the brain, use of the hands tends both to promote a feeling of psychological ease and to prevent hardening in the brain itself. The Chinese habit of turning walnuts round and round in the hand springs from a knowledge of the salutary effect of manual activity. Realizing that hotheads always lose, Japanese merchants, particularly drygoods dealers, long ago developed the practice of rubbing the hands together when dealing with trying customers because of the action's calming effect.

By putting the fingertips to extensive use, shiatsu promotes emotional stability and physical health as it stimulates the blood flow to the hands.

Correct Use of the Hands

a. Thumbs
Since the thumbs are often used in shiatsu treatment, they deserve careful attention. Always press downward firmly using the bulb of the thumb; never press forward with the tip because this can tire or perhaps injure your hands. Because living tissues develop as they are used, my forty-two years of correct shiatsu thumb action have given me well-developed, silky-smooth thumbs of the kind essential to my profession. Correct shiatsu can do the same for anyone *(Fig. 1)*.

b. Three Fingers
In treating the face and abdomen, employ the index, middle, and ring fingers *(Fig. 2)*.

c. Palm of the Hand
The palm of the hand is used to apply pressure to the eyes and abdomen and in vibration treatment.

Study the illustrations, and practice these basic methods carefully *(Fig. 3)*.

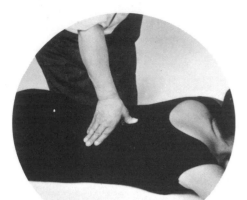

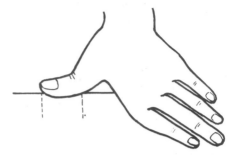

Fig. 1. Applying pressure with the thumb alone.

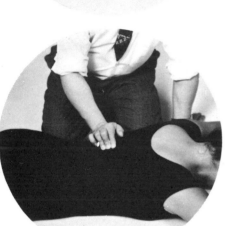

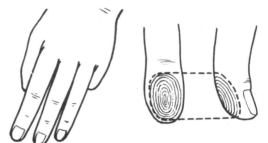

Fig. 2. Three fingers and bulb of the thumb.

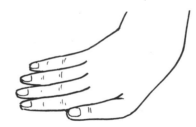

Fig. 3. Using the palm of the hand.

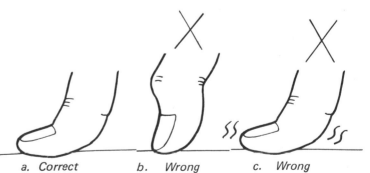

a. Correct   b. Wrong   c. Wrong

Fig. 4. Applying pressure.

Pressure is applied with the ball or the thumb straight down or with no rubbing motion.

Applying Pressure

Never jab your fingers into the flesh of the patient; instead apply firm pressure with the soft bulbs of the fingers or thumbs as if you were resting all your body weight on them. The degree of pressure needed depends on the symptoms and the personal condition, but your posture should always be such that, if necessary, you can apply your entire weight. The area of contact between the thumb and the body of the patient should be about the same as that inked on paper when fingerprints are taken. Pressure should be gentle and perpendicular to the area being treated.

Basic Pressure Points

Although certain points will need additional attention according to the nature of the patient's complaint, in general, to be effective, treatment must begin with applications of pressure on all the points illustrated in *(Fig. 5)*. To treat a specific illness, points nearest the ailing part demand attention, but sometimes pressure on distant areas brings greatest improvement: for instance, pressure on the soles of the feet for kidney disease and on the left hand to strengthen the heart. Experience proclaims the efficacy of shiatsu on apparently unrelated parts of the body, and factual medical bases substantiate it.

   All points of pressure are described later in full detail in sections arranged according to complaint.

Degree of Pressure

Except around the neck, where it must never exceed three seconds, the duration of a single application of shiatsu pressure should be from five to seven seconds. It should be sufficient to cause a sensation midway between pleasure and pain. A professional therapist can apply pressure that produces deep bodily effects without discomfort. Although, under clinical conditions, normally healthy patients usually undergo about thirty minutes of shiatsu treatment and invalids about one hour, the treatments described in this book require only three minutes each.

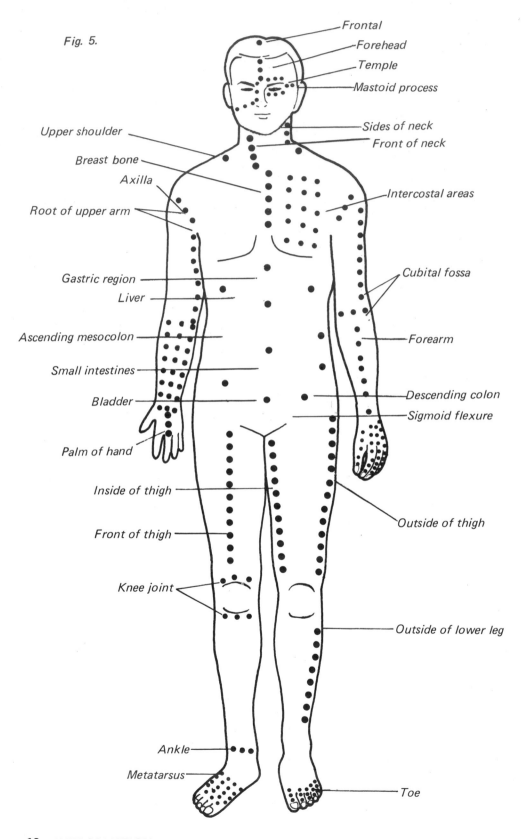

Fig. 5.

Frontal
Forehead
Temple
Mastoid process
Sides of neck
Front of neck
Upper shoulder
Breast bone
Axilla
Root of upper arm
Intercostal areas
Gastric region
Cubital fossa
Liver
Ascending mesocolon
Forearm
Small intestines
Bladder
Descending colon
Palm of hand
Sigmoid flexure
Inside of thigh
Front of thigh
Outside of thigh
Knee joint
Outside of lower leg
Ankle
Metatarsus
Toe

16   INTRODUCTION

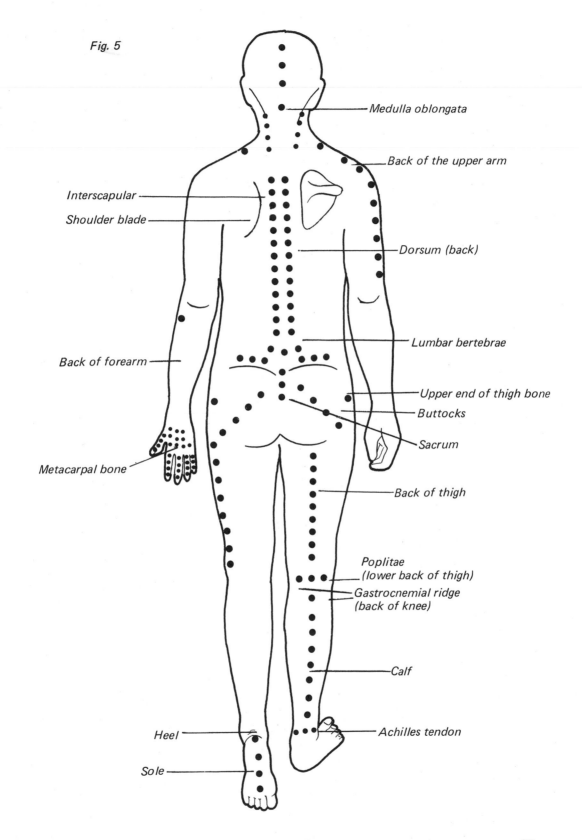

Fig. 5

Medulla oblongata

Back of the upper arm

Interscapular

Shoulder blade

Dorsum (back)

Lumbar bertebrae

Back of forearm

Upper end of thigh bone

Buttocks

Sacrum

Metacarpal bone

Back of thigh

Poplitae
(lower back of thigh)

Gastrocnemial ridge
(back of knee)

Calf

Heel

Achilles tendon

Sole

CHAPTER TWO

Better Health

Relief from Fatigue

If you awake every morning an hour or so before you must leave for work, feeling fit and clear headed—if you are a man, you will have a full erection, a symbol of health—you are one of the fortunate few leading reasonably comfortable, healthy, mentally and socially well adjusted lives. You have no cause to worry.

Modern city-dwelling working people, however, frequently lack sleep; after about three years on a job, they often become late-abed luggards whose wives or mothers find dragging them out in the morning an exasperating chore. Even the lucky people whose schedule permits lattitude of activity sometimes find that business, social, and home life creates tensions that manifest themselves as fatigue. The symptoms may take five, ten, or fifteen years to appear, and the person concerned may not recognize them even then; but we specialists know what is wrong at a glance.

To live a long, full life, a person must never allow fatigue to accumulate. During youth, eight hours of sleep usually wipe away all traces of fatigue; and even should exhaustion be severe, it often has no apparent lasting effect. However, drowsiness or languor in any part of the body indicates insufficient sleep and lingering fatigue. Such symptoms demand attention, for if unheeded they can lead to serious trouble.

What to Do When Weary

When your feet are tired, begin treatment by pressing each toe three times. Next press between the bones in the instep as if you were imprinting a thumbmark on the skin *(Fig. 6)*. After you have applied this pressure a few times, move on to the plantar arch (the sole of the foot), then to both the insides and outsides of the ankles and the Achilles tendon *(Fig. 7-9)*.

When fatigue is great, pressure on the plantar arch not only eliminates weariness, but also relieves ailments of the kidneys, with which it is closely related.

If time allows, continue applying pressure to the points from the ankle to the knee shown in *Figs. 10&11*. Begin at the

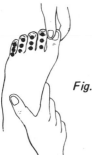

Fig. 6. Pressure points on the toe.

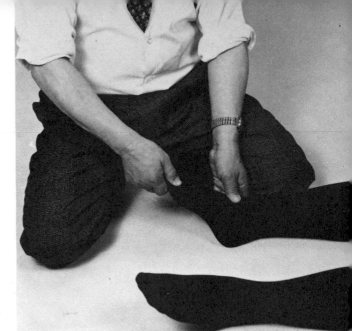

Fig. 7. The sole of the foot and the Achilles tendon.

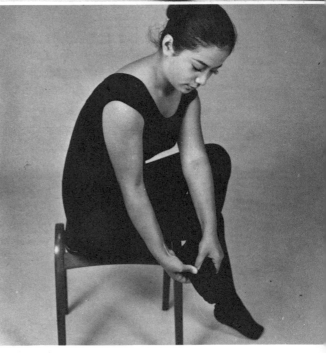

Fig. 8. Ankle.

Fig. 9. Heel.

Fig. 10. Knee.

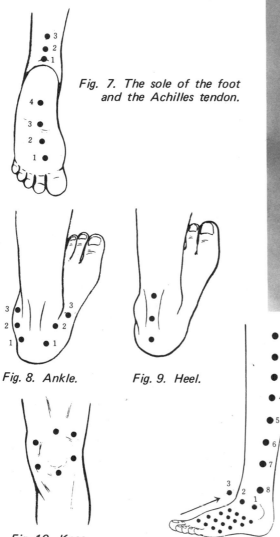

← sanri

Fig. 11. The topmost point is called the sanri. All the other points on the lower leg and foot require attention, time permitting.

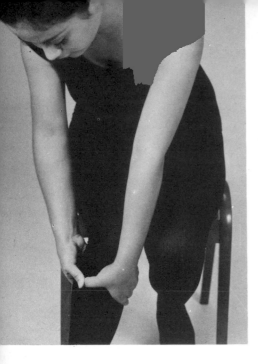

upper end of trochanter

trochanter majior

Fig. 13. Back of calf and knee.

calf

achilles tendon

Fig. 12. Hip and back of leg.

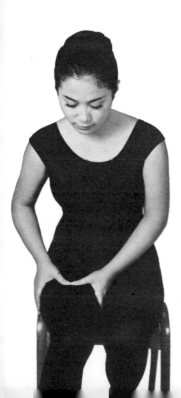

spot below the kneecap, called the *sanri* or three *ri* (literally, about 7.5 miles) because in ancient times, when practically all traffic in Japan was pedestrian, walkers weary from covering that distance sought relief by burning moxa on this part of the leg.

Continue by pressing the points from the *sanri* to the ankle and, with both thumbs, the points along the inside edge of the shin bone *(Fig. 12)*. Pinching the calf with five fingers *(Fig. 13)* relieves general fatigue and the sort of weariness caused by beriberi.

Shiatsu treatment of the thigh and groin aids in preserving youthfulness *(Fig. 14)*. Working downward, press the full length of the thigh muscle, first on the inside, then on the outside *(Figs. 15 & 16)* Next, using the four fingers of one hand, press the backs of the legs and the buttocks *(Fig. 12)*. Incidentally, withering of the flesh in the groin, particularly in young women, indicates a serious disorder, which should be corrected immediately.

Pressure on the sciatic nerve *(Fig. 17)* can prevent or cure neuralgia of the hip (ischianeuralgia). Apply shiatsu pressure to this nerve for about four minutes; then, lying on your back, stretch your arms straight above your head and against your ears and your legs straight and together. Extend your limbs three or four times as vigorously as possible.

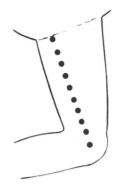

Fig. 14. Inside of thigh.

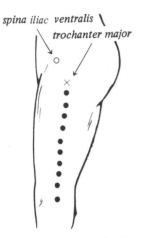

spina iliac ventralis
trochanter major

Fig. 15. Outside of thigh.

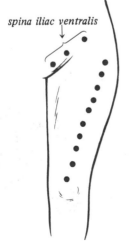

spina iliac ventralis

Fig. 16. Groin and inside of thigh.

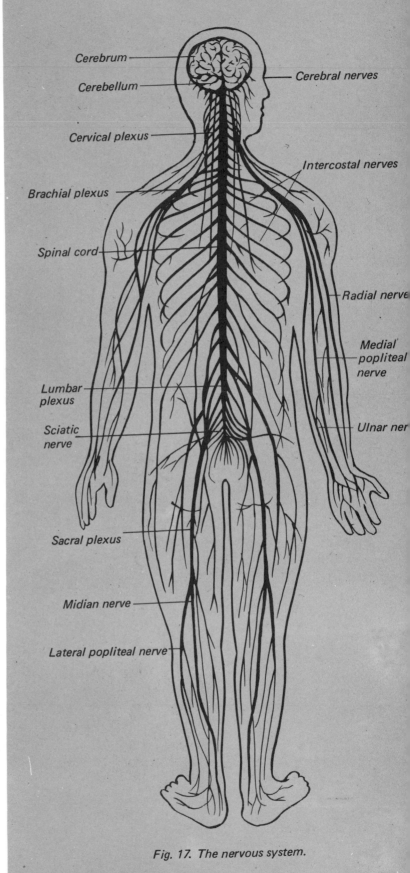

Cerebrum

Cerebellum

Cerebral nerves

Cervical plexus

Intercostal nerves

Brachial plexus

Spinal cord

Radial nerve

Medial popliteal nerve

Lumbar plexus

Sciatic nerve

Ulnar nerve

Sacral plexus

Midian nerve

Lateral popliteal nerve

Fig. 17. The nervous system.

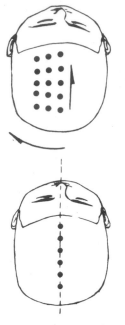

Fig. 18. Points to press on the crown of the head.

When the Head Feels Heavy

Long, late parties poison the following morning with hangovers. Everyone associated with the suffering victim feels the result of his intemperance in his short temper and sharp tongue. Actually, the cause of this complaint, stale, impure blood congested in the head area, can be eliminated quite easily by stimulating the flow of fresh blood with the following shiatsu treatment.

First, as you press your crown *(Fig. 18),* you will notice that your head begins to clear. Continue by using the bulb of the thumb to press first the right carotid artery and then the left lightly several times *(Fig. 19).* Begin at the jaw and work downward to the clavicle. This action causes the blood vessels to dilate so that they can bring fresh blood and consequently quick relief.

In addition to curing hangovers, shiatsu pressure applied to the head can relieve stiff necks and the mental fatigue that robs office workers of both efficiency and accuracy. Taking a few minutes to press the temples with three fingers *(Fig. 20)* or the back of the neck with four fingers and the nape of the neck with the thumbs *(Fig. 21)* restores alertness and energy and makes work easier.

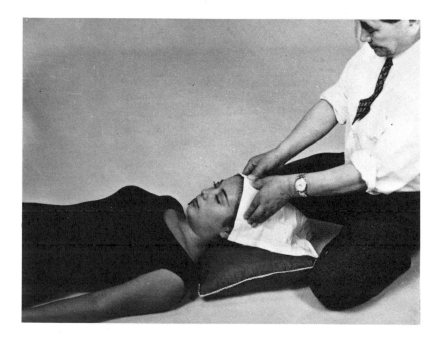

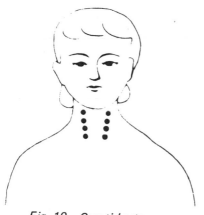

Fig. 19. Carotid artery

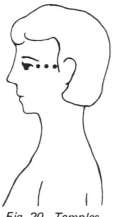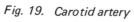

Fig. 20. Temples.

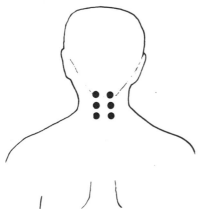

Fig. 21. Nape of the neck.

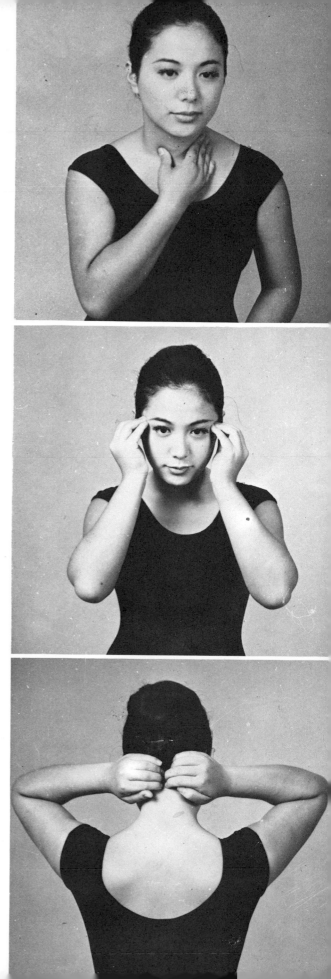

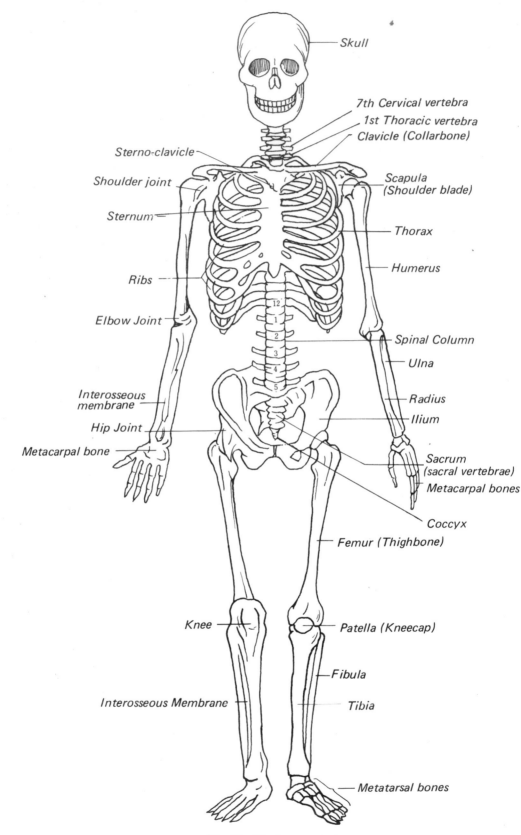

Skull

7th Cervical vertebra
1st Thoracic vertebra
Clavicle (Collarbone)

Sterno-clavicle

Shoulder joint

Scapula
(Shoulder blade)

Sternum

Thorax

Humerus

Ribs

Elbow Joint

Spinal Column

Ulna

Radius

Ilium

Interosseous
membrane

Hip Joint

Metacarpal bone

Sacrum
(sacral vertebrae)

Metacarpal bones

Coccyx

Femur (Thighbone)

Knee

Patella (Kneecap)

Fibula

Interosseous Membrane

Tibia

Metatarsal bones

12
1
2
3
4
5

Fig. 22. The human skeleton.

Fatigue of the Lower Back

Though people in their twenties know nothing about the feeling, aching, tired hips, the first signs of weariness accumulated over the years, demand immediate attention because this part of the body is the hub of such important movements as walking, stretching, leaning, and turning the trunk. Slouching produces an accumulation of fatigue in the loins, hardening of the back muscles, and disorders in the internal organs. Always take good care of the buttocks and hips, particularly if you are in your thirties; and if something goes wrong, try to correct it immediately. Chill, overwork, mental shock, dyskinesia caused by fever, or hernia of the invertebral discs cause serious lumbago; but slight, lumbago-like symptoms caused by sedentary work respond promptly to the following treatment. Firstly, always maintain an erect posture; secondly, when fatigue occurs, press with the thumbs along the lumbar and sacral vertebrae (*Fig. 23*).

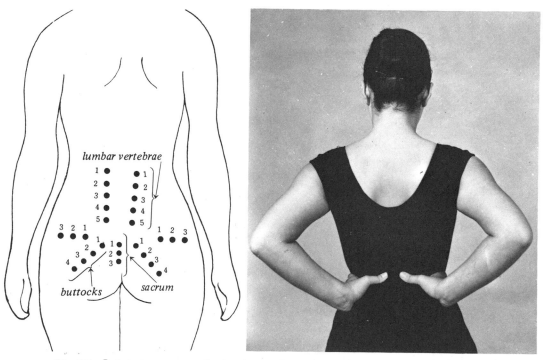

Fig. 23. *Points to press on the lumbar and sacral vertebrae, the sacrum, and the buttocks.*

Stiff Shoulders

Metabolic disturbances, diabetes, climateric disorders, or anemia may cause the sort of stiff shoulders that result in aching muscles in the shoulders and upper back (medically speaking, the trapezius, rhomboideus major, rhomboideus minor, and levator scapulae muscles), but the most ordinary causes are unnatural posture or irregularity of the spinal column or thoracic vertebrae. Should your shoulders become painfully stiff for no apparent reason, the following treatment usually relieves the strain that is almost always the cause.

Have a partner place both thumbs on your upper scapular region and resting his weight on them, press for three seconds, then release. He should repeat the application five or six times. Next have him press the points in the interscapular regions of the right and left shoulders three times (*Figs. 24&25*).

Putting the thumbs on the first point of the interscapular regions of both shoulders and the other fingers on the collarbones, your partner should apply pressure to all fingers simultaneously, squeeze the upper scapular muscle, and pull it upward. He should release after about one second; repeat three times.

Next, raising both your wrists, your partner should bend your body backward *(Fig. 26)*, release after three seconds, and drop your arms forward. After lifting both your upper arms and your shoulders three times *(Fig. 27)*, he should stroke your chest downward with the palms of his hand. Finally, he should stroke your spinal column downward lightly three times with the palm of his hand.

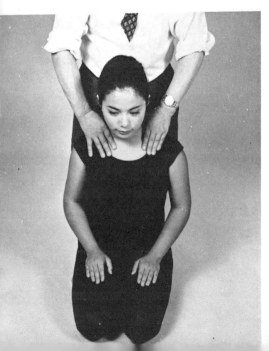

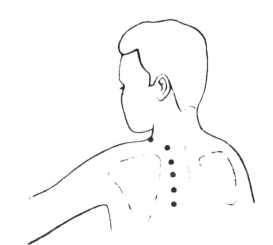

Fig. 24. Treating stiff shoulders. Point on top of shoulder, and interscapular region.

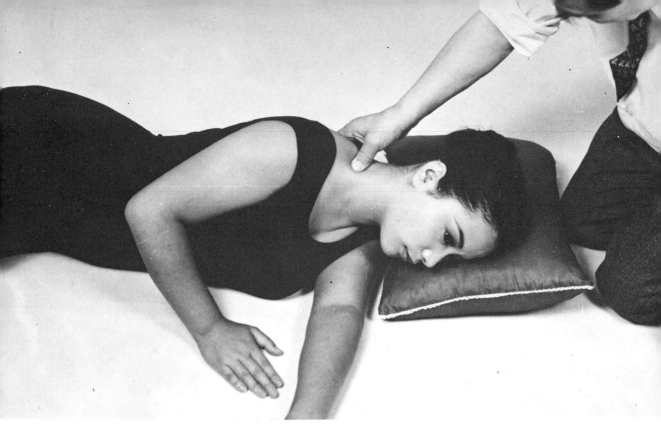

Fig. 25. Patient in a prone position.

26. Raising the patient's wrists and bending her body back.   Fig. 27. Lifting the patient's upper arms.

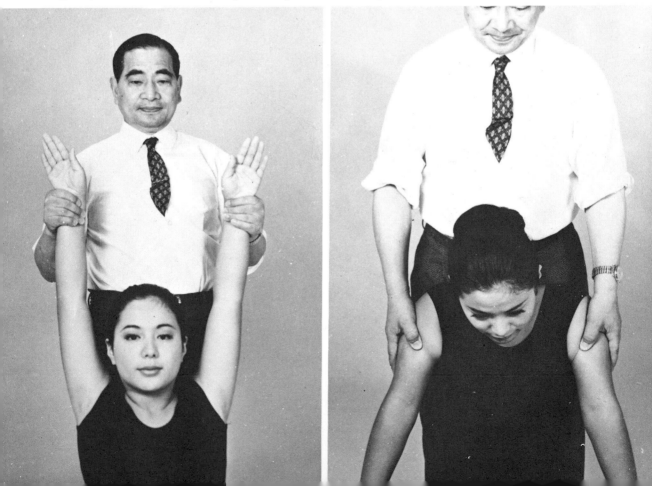

Tired Arms

A fire that has just started is easy to extinguish, whereas one that has been burning for some time may rage uncontrolled for days. The case is much the same with fatigue, easy to overcome if detected early but the cause of severe pain if allowed to accumulate. Pianists, typists, cashiers, key-punchers, accountants, or clerks obtain quick relief from sore arms and hands by applying shiatsu pressure to the points illustrated in *(Figs. 28–33).*

People employed as salesmen or in other occupations requiring prolonged standing or walking should emphasize shiatsu treatment of the feet and buttocks.

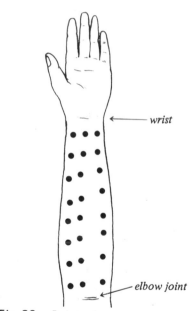

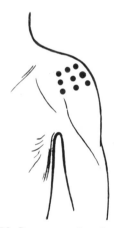

Fig. 29. *Pressure points in the area of the shoulder joint.*

Fig. 28. *Points for pressure from the elbow joint to the wrist.*

Fig. 30. *Outer side of the upper arm.*

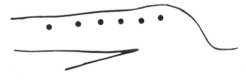

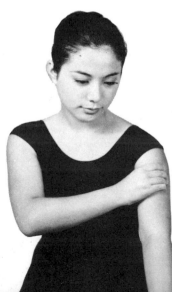

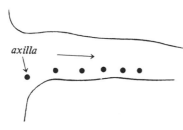

Fig. 31. Inner side of the upper arm.

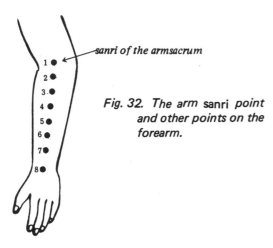

sanri of the armsacrum

1 ●
2 ●
3 ●
4 ●
5 ●
6 ●
7 ●
8 ●

Fig. 32. The arm sanri point and other points on the forearm.

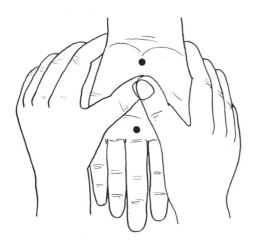

Fig. 33. Palm of the hand.

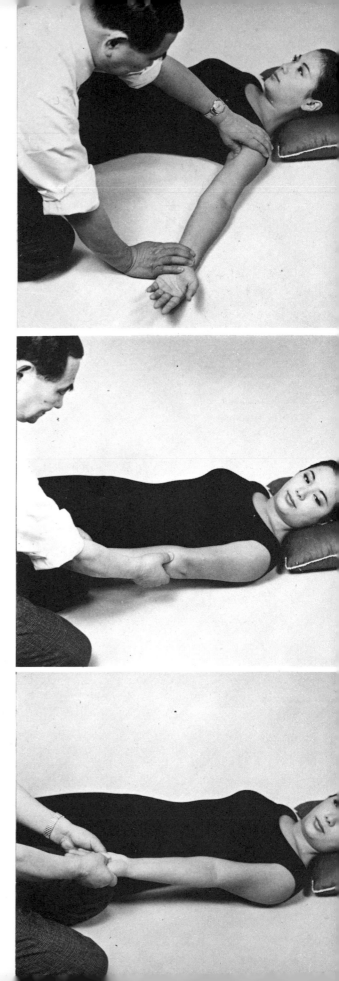

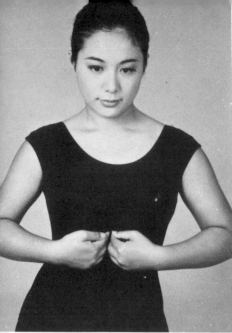

Fig. 34. *Applying pressure on the abdomen.*

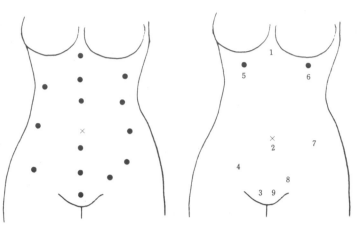

Fig. 35. *Pressure points on the trunk and in the abdominal area. 1. Stomach. 2. Small intestines. 3. Bladder. 4. Cecum. 5. Liver. 6. Spleen. 7. Descending colon. 8. Sigmoid flexure. 9. Rectum.*

Strengthening the Stomach

Loss of appetite often indicates a serious disorder in the body. To promote a hearty appetite, a sign of good health, apply shiatsu pressure to the abdominal region. By taking three minutes each morning before you arise to perform the following exercises you can help discharge gases that cause discomfort and, stimulating the flow of fresh blood into the area, thus improve metabolism. This treatment can help prevent ulcers, and even stomach cancer.

To apply the pressure to your own body, simply stretch your legs out, and press the index, middle, and fourth fingers of both hands into the pit of your stomach for about three seconds. Repeat three times. Moving a little farther down the abdomen, press three times, and still farther down, press three times again. Return to the starting point, and press three times on two points to the right and three times on two points to the left—that is, first over the spleen, then over the liver. Finally, placing the palm of the right hand over the gastric region and the left hand on the right hand, apply pressure for about thirty seconds; then release *(Fig. 34&35)*.

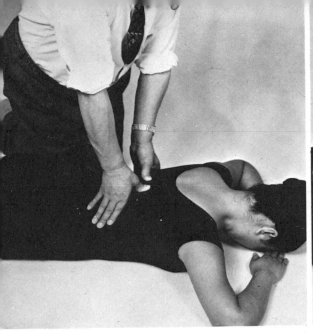

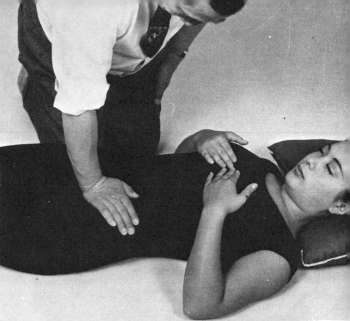

Fig. 36. *Treating a patient with a weak stomach.*
Fig. 37. *Stroking the abdomen.*

To perform shiatsu treatment on a person with a weak stomach, have him lie prone. Sitting to his right side, place both thumbs, one on top of the other, on the lumbodorsal fascia (fleshy area between the base of the left shoulderblade and the backbone). When the stomach is out of order this spot will be hard (*Fig. 36*).

Although the patient may complain at first, gradually the pain will subside. After pressing this point five or six times, press for about three seconds on each of nine points running from the left side of thorax (upper trunk) toward the buttocks. The points should be about one inch apart. Repeat the series three times; then perform it on the right side.

Having the patient lie on his back, sit at the right of his abdominal region, and stroke the pit of his stomach gently with the palm of the hand for about five seconds. Repeat five times. *Fig. 35* shows the points to press and the order in which to press them.

Since several important organs are located in the abdominal region, always use caution in applying pressure there. Should the patient complain of pain at any spot, an examination will usually reveal a lump at the location of the trouble; press gently to dissipate that lump *(Figs. 35—38).*

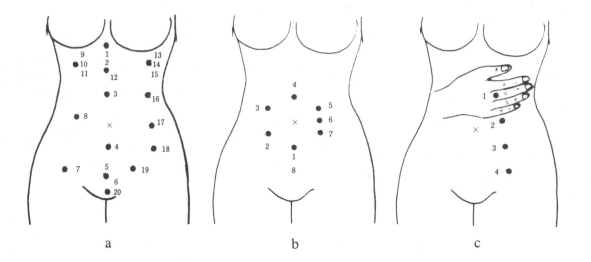

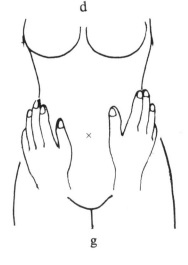

Fig. 38. A thorough abdominal treatment requires pressure on all these points.

a. Three applications with the fingers on each of these twenty points.

b. Three applications on each of these eight points on the small intestine.

c. Three applications with the palm of the hand on each of these four points on the descending colon.

d. Using the fingertips of both hands, placed on the navel, pull and press the descending colon.

  Applications of pressure in a circular motion cause vibration in the navel region.

e. Ten applications of pressure on the pelvis.

f. Ten applications with the fingers of both hands on the lumber vertebrae: the movement should suggest lifting the vertebrae.

g. Raise the abdomen three times, stroke it ten times, and cause vibration in the navel region.

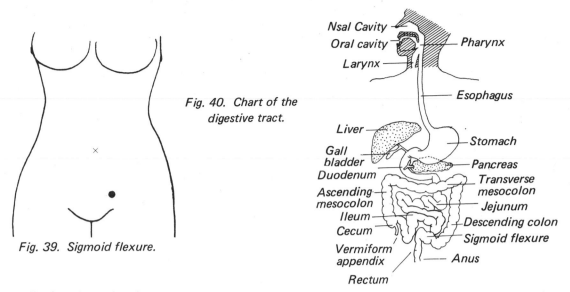

Fig. 40. Chart of the
digestive tract.

Nsal Cavity
Oral cavity
Larynx
Pharynx
Esophagus
Liver
Stomach
Gall
bladder
Pancreas
Duodenum
Transverse
mesocolon
Ascending
mesocolon
Jejunum
Ileum
Descending colon
Cecum
Sigmoid flexure
Vermiform
appendix
Anus
Rectum

Fig. 39. Sigmoid flexure.

Relieving Constipation

Elimination, one of the all-important bodily processes—digestion, assimilation, and elimination—is essential to good health.
To relieve chronic constipation, follow this routine every morning
before getting out of bed.

Feces tend to stagnate at an S-curve in the large intestine
located at the sigmoid flexure, diagonally left of the navel. A
chronically constipated person will have a lump at this spot. Using
the three-finger method *(p. 14)* in a rubbing motion, apply pressure with both hands to this area for about three minutes. Abdominal gurglings should begin, and you may feel the need to
evacuate. After drinking a glass of water with a little salt added,
go to the toilet. If you make this a daily morning routine, your
constipation will probably cease.

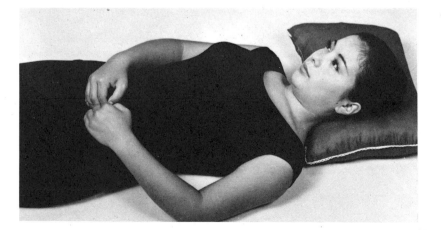

Sleeping Well

As the proverb goes, a baby that sleeps well grows fast, and certainly a good sleeper is usually a healthy person because slumber combats fatigue built up during the day. The amount of sleep needed depends on the individual and the degree of weariness, but generally speaking, six to eight hours are sufficient.

Napoleon—whether the legend of his sleeping only three hours a day is true or false—suggests two interesting points to the insomniac. He always said that, on retiring, he closed all the drawers in the cabinet of his brain and fell immediately into a sound sleep. To forget everything and sleep deeply, even for a little while, benefits the body much more than ten hours of wakeful, fitful tossing. Napoleon's second piece of good advice was to get up when you wake up. Lolling drowsily in bed for hours after profitable sleep has ended injures, rather than helps, for the body.

In addition to good mental advice, however, the insomniac sometimes needs physical therapy to induce the relaxation that will enable him to sleep well. The following procedure will help.

First, with the left thumb, press the left front of the neck *(Fig. 41)*, then along the carotid artery at four points leading to the clavicle. Repeat three times on the left and three times on the right side of the neck. Using the three-finger method *(P.14)*, press for three seconds on each of the three points over the medulla oblongata *(Fig. 42)*. Now press three points on the muscles along the back of the neck on both sides of the cervical vertebrae from the medulla oblongata to the tip of the shoulder. Repeat these three-second applications of pressure three times each.

Next, stretch out both legs, and point your toes first down, then up as far as possible to stimulate the flow of blood in the lower limbs; and finally, apply pressure with the bulbs of the fingers to the twenty points of the thorax *(p.34)*.

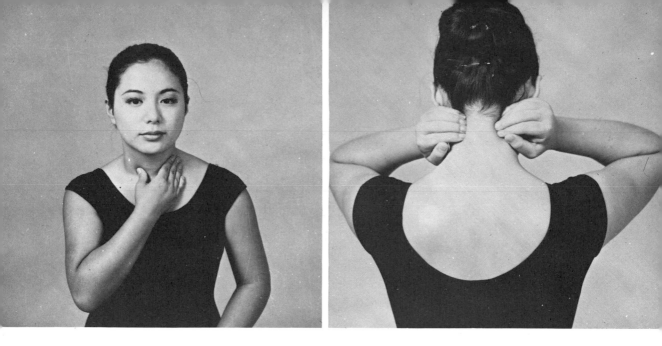

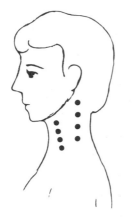

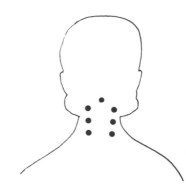

Fig. 41. Pressure points on the front and side of the neck.

Fig. 42. Pressure points for relief from insomnia.

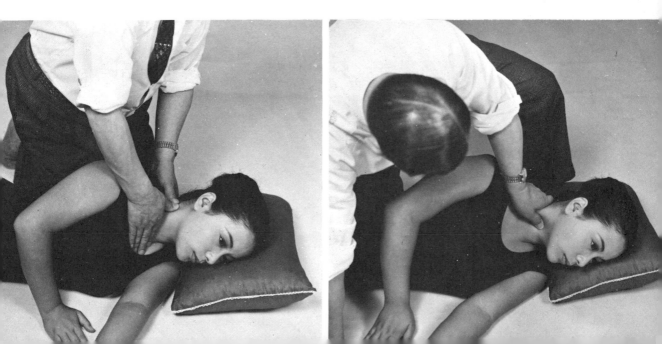

Strengthening the Internal Organs

Since the fingers are intimately connected with the internal organs—particularly with the brain—softening them and keeping them strong has a salutary effect on the total constitution.

People with heart trouble often have weak little fingers, sometimes to the extent that the finger will not straighten out properly. Conversely, exercising the little finger helps develop a stronger heart.

Similarly, shiatsu with the fourth finger helps cure liver trouble; and with the middle finger, high blood pressure and intestinal difficulties. Since people with weak index fingers often suffer from weak stomachs, a connection seems to exist between the two. People with strong thumbs tend to have powerful will because that finger influences the cerebrum.

Daily shiatsu with the fingers and as much manual exercise as possible help promote general health.

First, holding the left thumb between the thumb and index finger of the right hand and using a pulling motion, press on the three spots from the root to the tip, including the bulb *(Fig. 43).* Press first on the front and back and then on the sides of the thumb. The procedure with the other fingers is the same, except that, since they are longer, four pressure points are needed. Apply the same pressures to the fingers of the right hand.

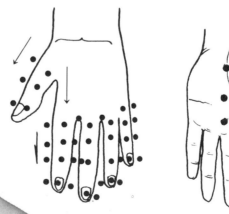

Fig. 43. Pressure points for developing strong hands.

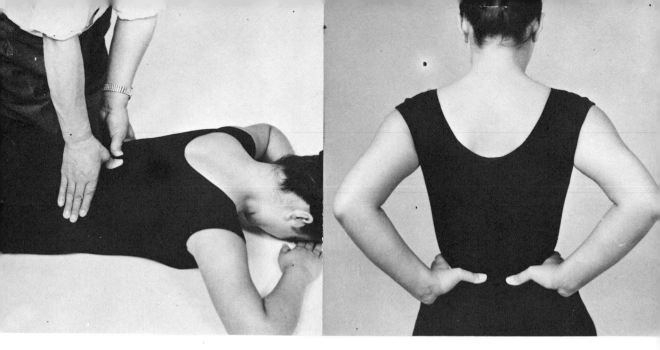

Developing Stamina

In the hectic, modern world, no one, no matter how intelligent or physically strong, succeeds without stamina. Although countless tonics proclaim stamina-giving powers, I am convinced that energy and strength need not necessarily come from a bottle. The shiatsu method, for instance, can work wonders.

Therapeutic pressure applied to the medulla oblongata affects the diencephalon, relieves stress, and stimulates the generation of stamina. A collection of nerve endings, located in the hollow of the nape of the neck, the medulla oblongata is the lowest part of the brain. It receives information from various parts of the body, forwards it to the nerve cells of other parts of the brain, and by doing so controls such important functions as swallowing, breathing, and the beating of the heart. So vital to life is this organ that a needle inserted into it immediately kills cats and dogs. Spanish matadors kill bulls by striking the medulla oblongata with their swords.

Producers of hormones, the adrenal glands, located near the eleventh and twelfth thracic vertebrae, also play an important part in developing stamina. To stimulate their action, apply shiatsu pressure to the sixth, seventh, and eighth points on both sides of the back (p. 17). For the sexual significance of these glands, see P. 50 .

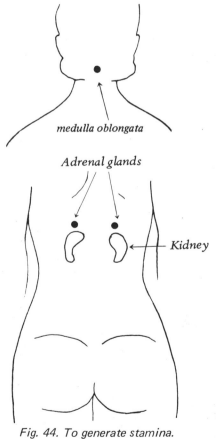

medulla oblongata

Adrenal glands

— *Kidney*

Fig. 44. To generate stamina.

The Liver

Pressing the area over the liver with one hand on top of the other ten times for three minutes each as you lie in bed in the morning helps promote stamina. The pain you may feel when you begin this treatment results from a liver disorder and should recede as shiatsu treatment brings about improvement. This method also helps prevent hangovers *(Fig. 45)*.

A good hearty laugh once a day stimulates action of the diaphragm which, in turn, activiates the digestive and respiratory systems. This, together with increased stamina, should keep a smile on your face all of the time.

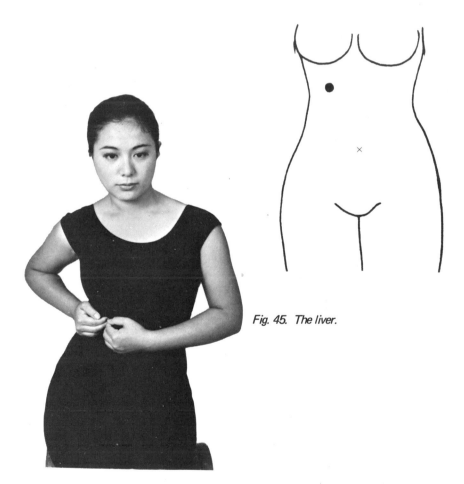

Fig. 45. The liver.

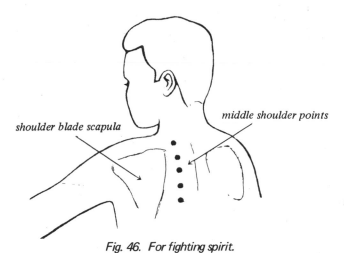

shoulder blade scapula

middle shoulder points

Fig. 46. For fighting spirit.

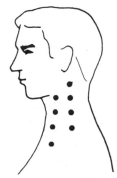

Fig. 47. Front and side of the neck.

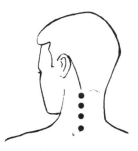

Fig. 48. Back of the neck.

Fighting Spirit

Shiatsu pressure on the roots of the shoulders and on the so-called middle-shoulder points *(Fig. 46)* creates the frame of mind necessary to the development of the will to win a sports competition, land a big contract, stay up all night to finish your tax forms, or do anything calling for extra fight power. To treat these points, press the thoracic vertebrae from right and left. You will require the assistance of another person, but only moderate pressure is needed.

Pressure on the neck also effects the generation of a fighting spirit. Using the left thumb, press the left front of the neck four times; use four fingers to press the back of the neck three times for each side. Next, place four fingers on the back of the head, and press the side of the neck with the bulbs of both thumbs three times for each of four points beginning below the ears. *(Figs. 47&48)*.

Lowering the High Blood Pressure

Lowering blood pressure and preventing arteriosclerosis, both important in reducing the danger of cerebral hemorrhage caused by erupting blood vessels in the brain, are accomplished by pressure applied to all parts of the body. Such thorough shiatsu keeps all of the muscles, consequently the blood vessels, flexible. The following exercises, however, are designed to supplement those directed toward total muscle tone.

With the bulb of the thumb, gently press the first point below the jaw (where pulse is felt) as you count to ten. Press, release, breathe, and press again. After repeating this three times on the left side, perform the same series three times on the right side. This spot *(Fig. 50)*, where the carotid arteries branch off, plays a role in adjusting blood pressure.

Next, using the middle fingers of both hands, press the medulla oblongata as you count to ten. Repeat three times *(Fig. 51)*.

Next, use three fingers of each hand to press the root of the occipital bone and three points above it. Increasing the pressure gradually each time, repeat three times *(Fig. 51)*. Press downward on both sides of the back of the neck with three fingers. Repeat three times for each of three points. Press three fingers of each hand into the pit of the stomach; count ten and release. Repeat ten times *(Fig. 52)*. Finally, apply a strong pulling pressure to the left middle finger, and then to the right middle finger *(Fig. 49)*.

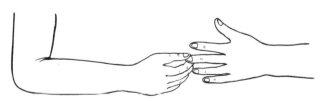

Fig. 49. Pulling the middle fingers.

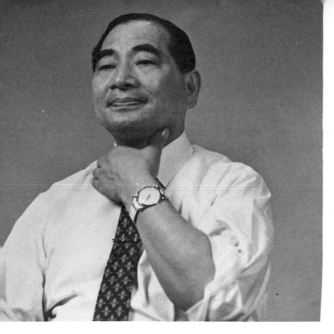

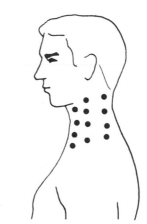

Fig. 50. Pressing the point below the jaw. Other points on the front and side of the neck.

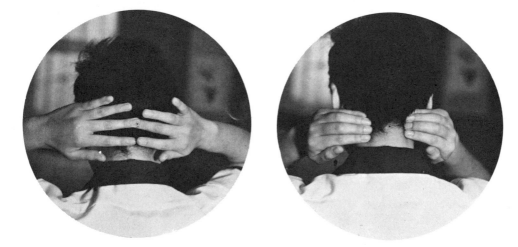

Fig. 51. The medulla oblongata and points on the back of the neck.

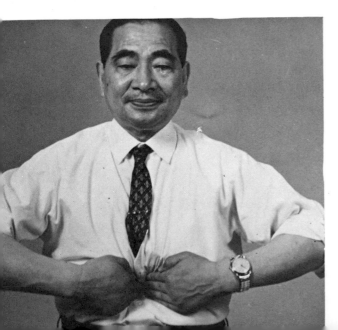

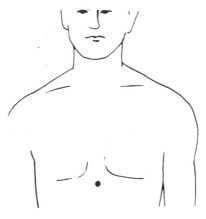

Fig. 52. The pit of the stomach.

Raising the Blood Pressure

Although blood pressures slightly lower than average are no cause for worry since they can even result in longer life, extreme low pressures, symptoms of cardiac weakness, can cause cerebral anemia. Any manifestation of such symptoms as excess fatigue, lassitude, dizziness, eye fatigue, insomnia, recurrent headaches, inability to concentrate, palpitation of the heart, short wind, or tightness in the chest or gastric region, requires an immediate check for low blood pressure.

These vague symptoms, often diagnosed as neurosis or slight anemia, as well as the so-called dizzy spells (orthostatic hypotensive asthenia) caused by rising suddenly or attempting to lift something heavy indicate malfunctions in the autonomous nerve system controlling blood pressure. To correct the difficulty, press first on the carotid sinus, then on the back of the head, the area above the medulla oblongata, the upper shoulder, and the space between the shoulder blades. (Fig. 53).

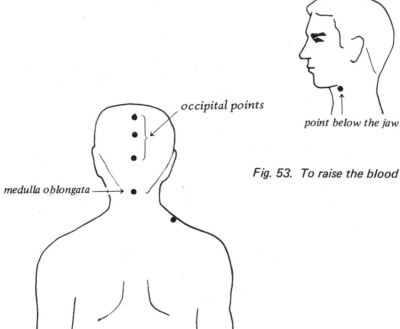

occipital points

point below the jaw

medulla oblongata

Fig. 53. To raise the blood pressure.

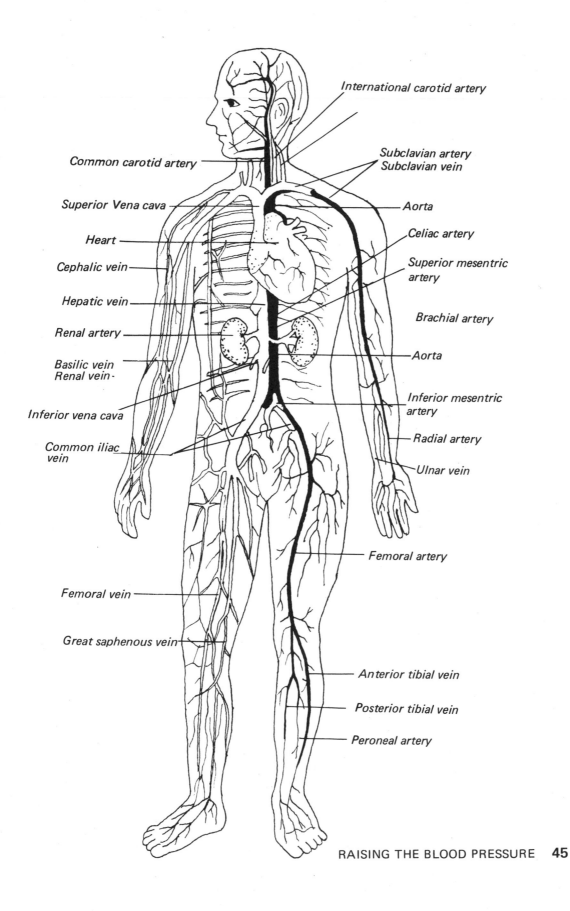

International carotid artery

Subclavian artery
Subclavian vein

Common carotid artery

Aorta

Celiac artery

Superior Vena cava

Superior mesentric
artery

Heart

Cephalic vein

Brachial artery

Hepatic vein

Renal artery

Aorta

Basilic vein
Renal vein

Inferior mesentric
artery

Inferior vena cava

Radial artery

Common iliac
vein

Ulnar vein

Femoral artery

Femoral vein

Great saphenous vein

Anterior tibial vein

Posterior tibial vein

Peroneal artery

Strengthening the Heart

The stress of modern living often causes palpitations of the heart, short wind, discomfort around the heart, and sometimes pain and other symptoms resembling cardiac disorder when the patient, in fact, suffers from none of the organic ailments: valvular heart disease or cadiac infarction weakness. These neurotic symptoms, caused by imbalance in the vasomotor center below the hypothalamus in the midbrain, disturb circulation throughout the body, affect the heart itself, and by confusing the nerve centers in the hypothalamus create short wind, fever, and perspiration. Because the midbrain is the relay station for all of the senses, naturally, emotional stresses on it affect the heart also. Conversely, since the state of the heart controls the senses, any disturbance in that organ, even a neurotic one, creates anxieties which only aggravate the upset in the midbrain.

The best way out of this vicious circle is to avoid mental and physical overwork, late hours, stimulating foods and drinks, and tobacco and to lead a well regulated life. Once the symptoms appear, however, they can be relieved by shiatsu pressure on the head, forearms, medulla oblongata, shoulder blades (especially the left one), the area from the breast to the armpits, and the pit of the stomach. Using the palms of the hands, press deeply and gently *(Fig. 55, a~f)*.

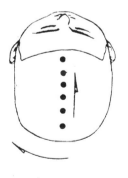

a. Center line of the crown.   *b. Underside of the forearm.*

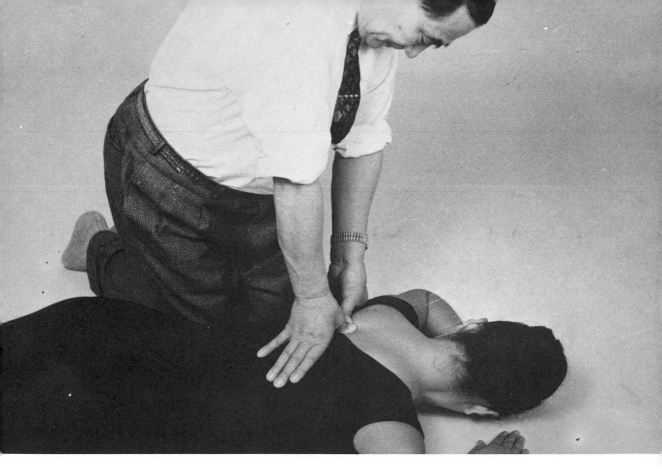

Fig. 55. Strengthening the heart.

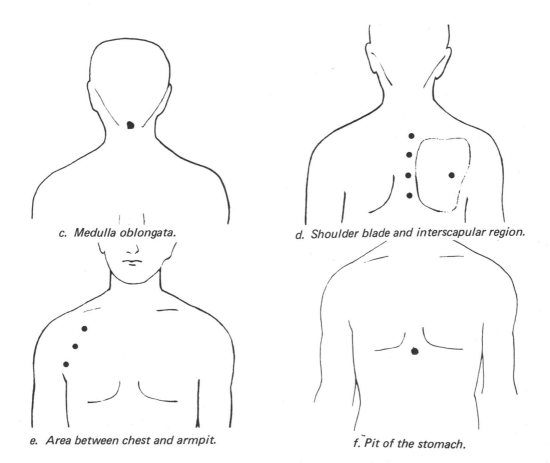

c. Medulla oblongata.

d. Shoulder blade and interscapular region.

e. Area between chest and armpit.

f. Pit of the stomach.

CHAPTER THREE
Sex-related Shiatsu

A Healthful Sex Life

The following shiatsu routines can help increase sexual pleasure and thereby promote happier marital relations.

Improving Sexual Performance in the Male

The sacrum

To prevent loss of sexual energy, apply shiatsu pressure to the lumbar region, where the genital nerves are concentrated. Lightly pressing the points at the sacral vertebrae, in the small of the back between the waist and the coccyx, ten times for three seconds each strengthens these nerves, even in middle-aged golfers, who sometimes suffer injuries in this region and, consequently, complain of dwindling potency.

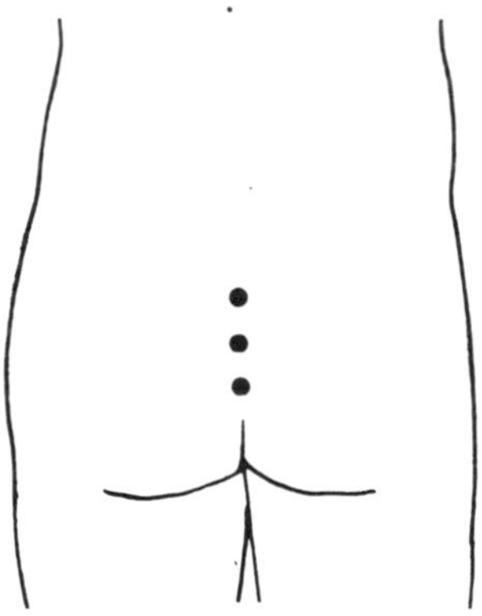

Fig. 56. Three points at the sacral vertebrae.

The pit of the stomach
Pressing the pit of the stomach with three fingers (ten times, five seconds each) vitalizes the lumbar region and aids in promoting sexual energy.

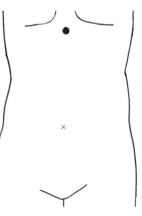

Fig. 57. The pit of the stomach.

The liver

Liver ailments, common among office workers, decrease sexual potency, but frequent pressure applied to the area just below the right rib will bring relief.

Incidentally, anger, as the Chinese proverb says, is bad for the liver; therefore, it limits sexual enjoyment.

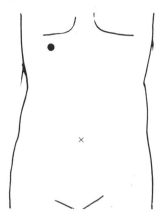

Fig. 58. Pressure applied over the liver.

Relieving constipation

By opposing a building up of energy, constipation weakens all human activities, including sex. For relief, gently knead the area left of the navel over the sigmoid flexure.

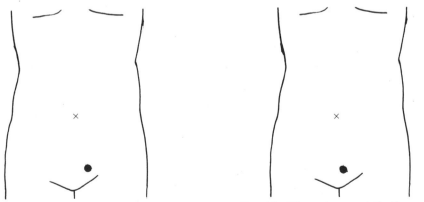

Fig. 59. Point over the sigmoid flexure   *Fig. 60. The pubo-prostatic ligament.*

The bladder

Pressure on the area between the navel and the gastric region stimulates the bladder and, consequently, sexual response. Rubbing the pubo-prostatic ligament, located at the border of the public hair, increases sensitivity in the testicles.

Anal and Perineal Regions

Firm pressure first around the anus and then on the perineal area, between the anus and the genitals, stimulates sexual response.

The testicles

Squeezing the testicles firmly—the Japanese proverb says once for every year of your life—proves particularly invigorating as one grows older.

Premature Ejaculation

Although, in some cases, young, inexperienced men ejaculate prematurely, other men with more than sufficient experience, when bombarded by the too abundant sexual stimuli of our age, are unable to perform adequately at the proper time. Frequent shiatsu pressure applied to the pit of the stomach and the sacrum should relieve the difficulty.

This same exercise will assist men of more than fifty years of age in performing the sexual act several times with only one ejaculation: loss of large amounts of sperm is fatiguing.

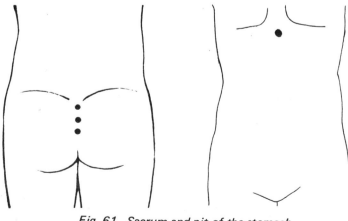

Fig. 61. Sacrum and pit of the stomach.

Increasing Sexual Ability in the Female

In addition to those mentioned in the many sexology books on the market, I have discovered a number of points on the female body where shiatsu pressure on endocrine glands and sensitive spots stimulates sexual response.

Thyroid gland — In front of the neck above the clavicle.

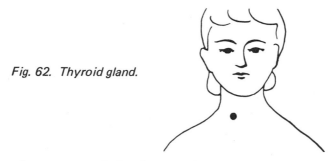

Fig. 62. Thyroid gland.

Area above to the suprarenal gland — Apply pressure to those points with the fist.

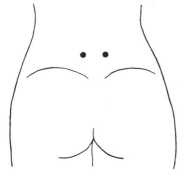

Fig. 63. Suprarenal glands.

Between the breasts — An endocrine gland is located here.

Fig. 64. Endocrine gland between the breasts.

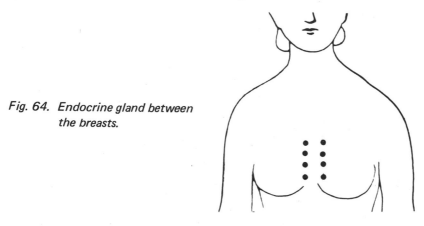

Inguinal regions — Insides of the thighs. (*Fig. 65*)

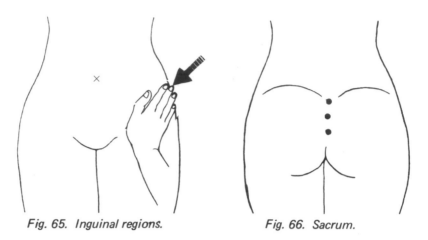

Fig. 65. *Inguinal regions.*   Fig. 66. *Sacrum.*

Sacrum — Pressing this area on the female produces much the same effect as on the male *(Fig. 66)*.

Curing Frigidity

1. The woman should lie on her stomach.
2. Working downward, with all your weight press both sides of the third, fourth, and fifth lumbar vertebrae—the fifth lumbar vertebra is at waist level.
3. Next, gently press the points on the buttocks *(Fig. 67)*.
4. Finish with a thorough shiatsu treatment of the front of the neck (over the thyroid gland), the tender spot at the medulla oblongata, the breasts, and the insides of the thighs.

Satisfying sex manifests itself in a well-ordered, total way of life, and shiatsu, practiced by man and wife, not just in the bedroom, but whenever the occasion arises, plays a large part in keeping marital sex thrilling.

Fig. 67. *Fifth lumbar vertebrae. Points on the lumbar vertebrae, sacrum, and buttocks.*

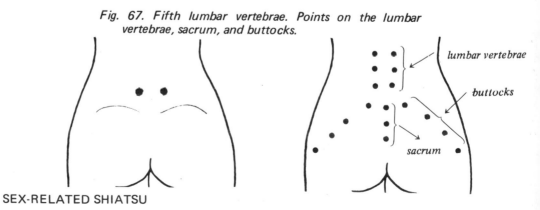

lumbar vertebrae

buttocks

sacrum

Pressure on the Thyroid Gland

Pressing the ductless, or endocrine glands, keeps the skin beautiful and the face and figure, charming by stimulating the production of hormones. More than four thousand years ago, the ladies of an Indian harem, though ignorant of medical science, learned by instinct that pressure on the thyroid helped them stay lovely enough to keep the attention of the king.

To do the same, all that is necessary is to bend your neck slightly forward and press the bulb of your left thumb into the fourth neck point (the area above the thyroid gland). Press gently for two seconds; release. Repeat five times on the left, then five times on the right side with the right thumb. Perform the entire series, left and right, three times. Practiced often, this exercise can also prevent hair from turning gray. Doing it in the bath is a good idea.

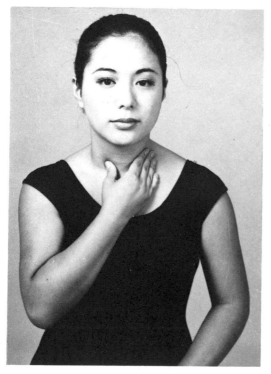

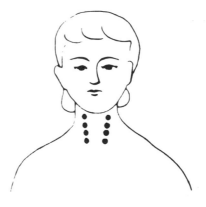

Fig. 68. Pressing the thyroid glands to beautify the skin.

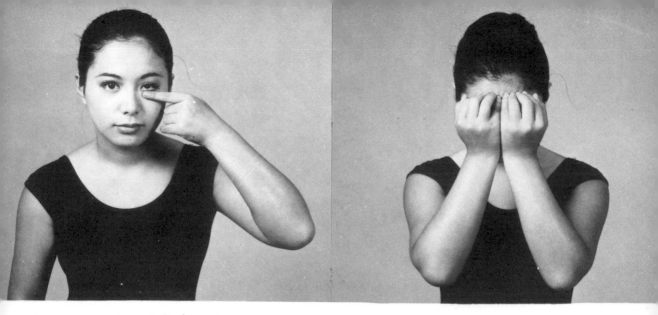

Fig. 69. Pressure points for improving the appearance of the eyes and for relief of eyestrain.

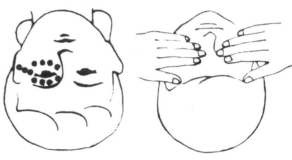

Beautifying the Eyes

To keep your eyes bright, clear, and appealing and to obtain quick relief from eye pain, headaches, and heaviness or pressure in the head brought on by close work, reading, or too much television, follow this routine.

1. Press upward three times under the eyebrow along the eye socket with three fingers. Do not let the fingernails touch the skin.

2. Next press downward three times on the lower part of the socket.

3. Finally, apply pressure to the eyelids with the bulbs of the thumbs for about ten seconds. A thorough shiatsu treatment of the face completes the series *(Fig. 69)*.

You might, however, if time allows, press three fingers against the nose near the temple (trigeminal nerves) and on the temples themselves. If this is not enough to relieve your condition, apply pressure to the area between the superior angle and the medial border of the shoulder blades.

Enlarging the Breasts

The most effective shiatsu course to achieve this effect consists of pressure on the thyroid gland, medulla oblongata, the upper shoulder, middle shoulder, and finally the breasts, where a kneading massage with the palms not only enlarges the breasts, but also helps them keep their shape.

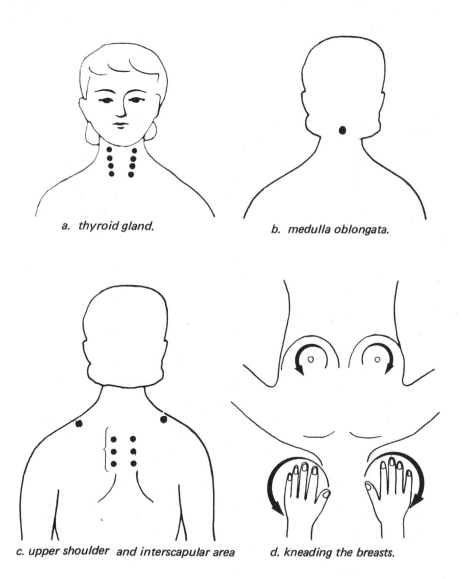

a. thyroid gland.

b. medulla oblongata.

c. upper shoulder and interscapular area

d. kneading the breasts.

Fig. 70. Pressure applied to the eyelids.

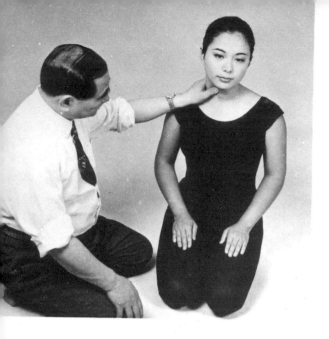

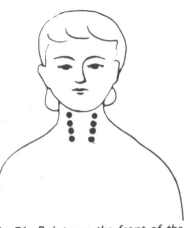

Fig. 71. Points on the front of the neck over the thyroid gland.

Climacteric Troubles (Menopause)

A natural phenomenon, like morning sickness during pregnancy, change of life is unavoidable; but its course depends on physical constitution, childbirth experience, number of children born, and nutritional elements. It usually begins with irregular menstruation, which may cease within a few months or last for years. As the ovaries shrink, development of the ovum and ovulation become irregular and finally stop altogether. Hot flashes and neurosis plus several symptoms of age, brought on by disorders and imbalances in the ductless glands (especially the anterior lobe of the hypophysis, thyroid, and suprarenal glands and the pancreas) and malfunctions of the autonomic nerves controlling them, usually accompany menopause. Tenseness in the sympathetic and parasympathetic nervous systems brings about disturbances in the motor nerves, dizziness, palpitations, sweating, hysteria, ringing in the ears, climacteric high blood pressure, increased or decreased pulse rate, flushed face, hot flashes, loss of appetite, change of tastes, stubborn diarrhea or constipation, moodiness, excitability, melancholia, heaviness in the head, chronic headache, insomnia, or lapses of memory.

   To solve some of the problems, apply shiatsu pressure in the following way.

1. Begin by pressing the front of the neck (particularly at the fourth point over the thyroid).

2. Go on to press the medulla oblongata, upper shoulder, middle shoulder, abdomen, pit of the stomach, and lower abdomen.

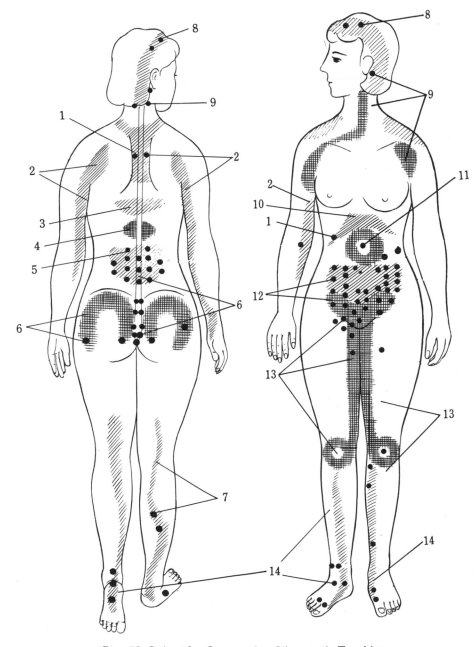

Fig. 72. Points for Overcoming Climacteric Troubles

1. *3rd to 5th thoracic vertebrae, middle shoulder*
   (effective for palpitation, stiff shoulders)
2. *Clavicle and inside of the upper arm*
   (gastric region, female organs)
3. *6th to 8th thoracic vertebrae and on both sides*
   (stomach, liver)
4. *10th to 11th thoracic vertebrae and on both sides*
   (suprarenal gland, hysteria)
5. *Lumbar region*
   (kidneys, abdominal region, reproductive organs)
6. *3rd to 5th lumbar vertebrae, sacral vertebrae, buttocks*
   (sexual glands)
7. *Median line of the calf, popliteal fossa*
   (nerve disturbances)
8. *Parietal fossa, front of the neck, armpit, cubital fossa*
   (reproductive organs, autonomic nerves, thyroid gland)
9. *The neck*
   (gall-bladder, bladder, hypophysis cerebri)
10. *Precordial depression, intercostal arch*
    (stomach, liver)
11. *Gastric region*
    (hysterial)
12. *Around the navel, small intestine*
    (internal organs)
13. *Abdominal region, inguinal region, inside the thingh*
    Abdominal region, inguinal region, inside the thighs, knee
    (female organs)
14. *Front of the leg, ankle, instep, sole*
    (gall bladder, stomach, liver)

CHAPTER FOUR

Shiatsu Treatment of Specific Illnesses

Gastralgia

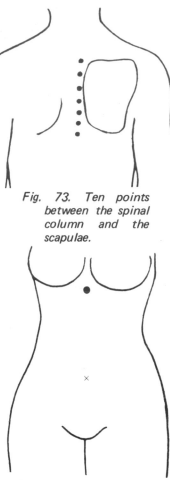

Fig. 73. Ten points between the spinal column and the scapulae.

Fig. 74. The pit of the stomach.

Sudden and acute pains in the stomach usually mean gastritis, most of the causes of which are nervous. If the pain is on the right side or in the pit of the stomach, it could be a disorder of the gall bladder.

1. To bring about quick relief of gastralgia, have the patient lie on his stomach.
2. Straddle his body, and place your right thumb on the fifth point between the shoulder blades *(Fig. 75)*.
3. Put the left thumb on top of the right one, and press with the full weight of your body for five seconds. Repeat five or six times.
4. If the patient still complains of pain, apply pressure to his spine along the sides of the vertebrae from about one inch below the fifth point down to the fifth lumbar vertebra. Apply the pressure for five or six times for three seconds each *(Fig. 73)*.
5. Next have him turn over on his back, and press the pit of his stomach lightly with the palm of your right hand. After five or six minutes of this treatment, he should sleep comfortably *(Fig. 74)*

Incidentally, I once brought great relief to the late motion-picture idol Marylin Monroe when she and her husband Joe di Maggio were on their honeymoon in Tokyo. Miss Monroe, then in the prime of her great beauty, was suffering from an attack of spasms of the stomach. I administered shiatsu treatment, which was a complete success.

Fig. 75. Quick relief from gastralgia.

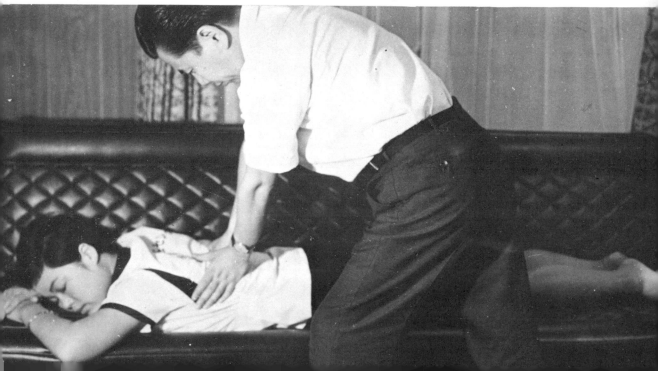

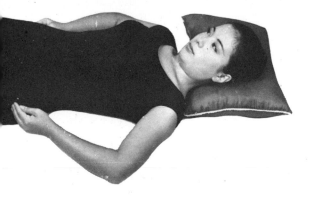

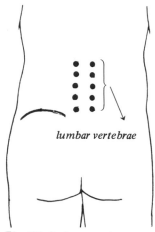

Fig. 76. Points on the scapula.

Diarrhea

Excess peristaltic action of the small intestine, characteristic of diarrhea, results from extraordinary stimulus to the intestinal wall, heightened sensitivity of the intestinal mucous membrane, or malfunction of the autonomic nerves controlling peristaltic activity. Less severe cases of diarrhea may, however, be caused by indigestion from overeating or excessive drinking, stimulation from accumulated excrement, psychogenic diarrhea (often the result of strain), food allergies, gastrogenic diarrhea (the result of a shortage of digestive fluid), nocturnal chill, or the common cold. The more serious forms of the ailment, brought on by enteritis, contagious diseases—dysentery or cholera—tuberculosis, ulcerative colitis, rectal cancer, abnormalities in glandular secretion resulting from thyroid disease, Addison's disease, or toxins produced by pneumonia, septicemia, and toxicosis require the immediate attention of a physician.

lumbar vertebrae

Fig. 77. Points on the small of the back at either side of the spinal column.

On the other hand, to obtain relief from diarrhea caused by impediments in the reflex nervous system, follow this shiatsu routine.

1. Apply pressure to the areas closest to the midbrain and the back of the head: these control the reflex nervous system (Fig. 73).
2. Press the points around the scapulae and the armpits to produce a stiffening in the muscle from the scalpulae on both sides at the points that play an important role in strengthening the stomach and intestines. (Fig. 76).
3. Press the small of the back and, more important, the sacrum.
4. Apply pressure to the hip points up to the trochanter major: these are the key points in treating diarrhea (Fig. 77).
5. Using the thumbs, apply considerable pressure to the point between the bases of the big and second toes. Five or six applications on each foot should suffice. (Fig. 78).
6. Finally, press the area over the descending colon and the lower abdomen lightly and gently with the palm of the hand.

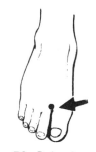

Fig. 78. Point between the bases of the big and second toes.

Gastroptosis (Fallen Stomach)

People whose work requires them to stand or sit for long periods in one position—drivers, beauticians, barbers, teachers, etc.—are often pale and thin as a result of a condition called gastroptosis, or fallen stomach. Usually overeating or excessive use of medicines and digestives, or sometimes a congenital weakness of the supporting muscles, causes the lower section of the stomach to fall to the level of the umbilicus or, in severe cases, to the pelvis, where it exerts enough pressure to displace other internal organs. In women, the condition produces an accompanying drooping of the ovaries and the uterus.

Patients suffering from gastroptosis usually complain of a heavy, distended stomach, loss of appetite, fatigue, dizziness, headache, and loss of weight. They are often nervous, fidgety people, who cherish their illnesses.

The first thing to remember in curing gastroptosis is to assure your patient that cure is possible and to put his mind at rest. Follow this with admonitions to improve his general physical condition, and finally employ shiatsu to strengthen the abdominal muscles and peritoneum. In most instances, it is also important to institute treatment to restore the total functions of the stomach in order to cure the dyspepsia and constipation often accompanying gastroptosis.

Other areas requiring attention are the shoulders and neck, which, in nervous moody people are often stiff and hard, and the chest, where knot-like muscular swellings sometimes occur above the pectoralis major (large chest muscle). These knots should be rubbed forcibly but gently.

To promote general health and accelerate the cure of gastroptosis, apply pressure to the following points for the reasons given.

1. Points six, seven, and eight of the thoracic vertebrae and surrounding tissue—to treat stomach and liver *(Fig. 79)*.
2. Points nine through twelve of the thoracic vertebrae and surrounding tissue—to strengthen the kidneys.
3. Points on the suprarenal gland, the shoulder blades, upper back near the armpits, latissimus dorsal muscle (lower part of back), and forearm—to dispel neurotic symptoms.
4. Point four of the lumbar vertebrae, the buttocks, the front

of the thigh, the calf, and the front of the neck — to stimulate the pneumogastric nerve (*Figs. 80–82*).

The final and most difficult phase of the course, treating the abdomen, requires light pressure with the palm of the hand over the epigastric region (stomach). To restore the stomach to its correct location, push upward carefully from the umbilicus to the lower abdomen. Never use force. Continue the treatment by applying light pressure to the inguinal region (the groin where the abdomen joins the thighs) and, with the thumbs, to the sanri to relieve fatigue and chill, both symptomatic of gastroptosis.

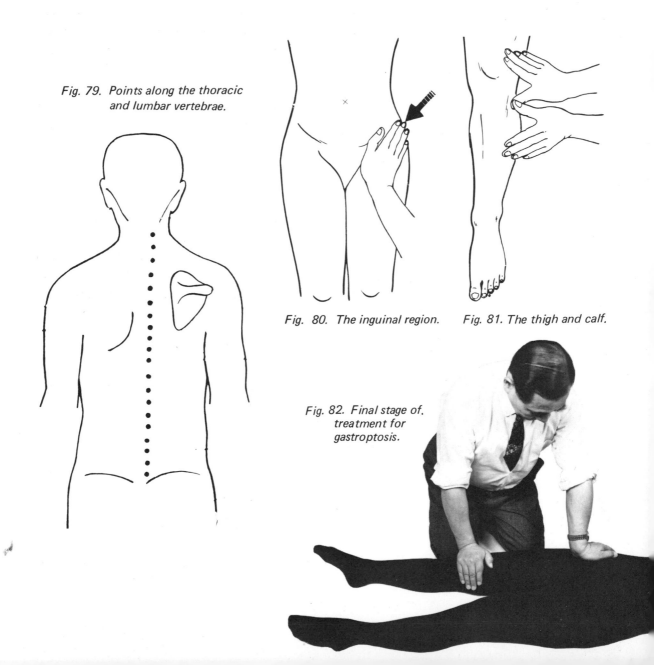

Fig. 79. Points along the thoracic and lumbar vertebrae.

Fig. 80. The inguinal region.

Fig. 81. The thigh and calf.

Fig. 82. Final stage of treatment for gastroptosis.

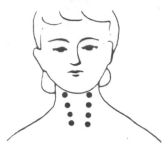

Fig. 83. Points on the front of the neck.

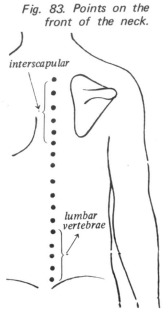

Fig. 84. Points on the thoracic and lumbar vertebrae.

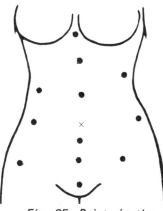

Fig. 85. Points in the abdominal region.

Common Cold

Practically no one can escape the common cold, which comes upon us when body heat fails to adjust to skin temperature, as when, during sleep, the body lowers its internal temperatures while expanding the capillaries supplying the skin. Because the resulting imbalance leaves the body vulnerable to colds, proper covering at night is of great importance, even during the summer months. Naturally, however, constitution and powers of resistance largely determine an individual's degree of vulnerability.

The head cold, characterized by coryza, laryngitis, and sore throat, is less a disease than an alarm signal indicating the body's inability to adjust to its environment or to resist possible virus infections. To cope with this problem, shiatsu treatment raises the resistance of the entire body instead of attempting to treat specific organs. Nevertheless, shiatsu pressure on the front of the neck, upper shoulders, interscapular region, lower back, lower legs, thighs, and abdomen relieves a cold's unpleasant symptoms (Fig. 83–85).

Nasal Congestion

1. Press firmly on the front of the neck.
2. Next, using the middle finger placed on top of the index finger, apply repeated pressure to both sides of the nose from the root to the nostrils. This should clear up the congestion quickly. Although it is possible to use the middle finger alone, in self-shiatsu, the combination of two fingers increases the treatment's effectiveness (Fig. 86).

Hoarseness

1. Press repeatedly on the third and fourth points in the front of the neck.
2. Apply gentle shiatsu pressure to the occipital region, the upper shoulder, and the solar plexus (pit of the stomach).

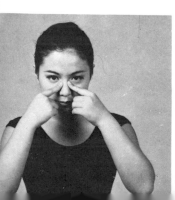

Fig. 86. Clearing nasal congestion.

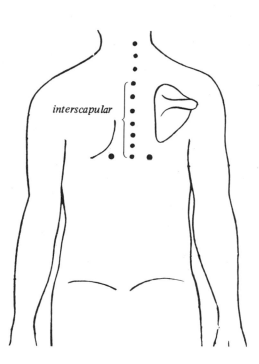

interscapular

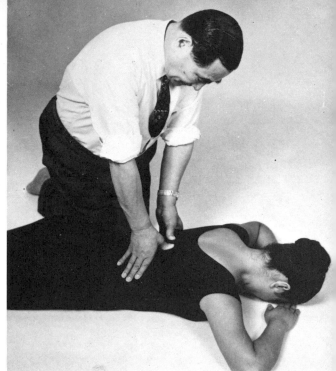

Fig. 87. The seventh cervical vertebra.

Diabetes

This disease, on the increase among the young as well as the elderly, causes both sexual impotency and fatigue that interferes with daily activities. Resulting from the failure of the pancreas to secrete sufficient insulin and a consequent escape of sugar into the blood stream, diabetes is ordinarily treated with injections of insulin taken from the pancreases of cattle. Although this therapy alleviates the symptoms, it no more solves the problem than borrowing water from a neighbor will make a man's own well full again. Shiatsu pressure on key points, however, can help the pancreas renew its important functioning.

1. Have the patient lie on his stomach, and feeling along the back of the neck, locate the seventh cervical vertebra, the most prominent in the series. Count ten vertebrae down from the seventh cervical, and you should locate stiff hard muscle on either side of the spine. This muscle must relax in order to improve the functioning of the pancreas *(Figs. 87&88).*

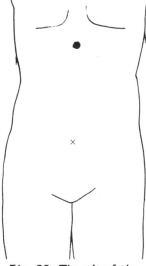

Fig. 88. The pit of the stomach.

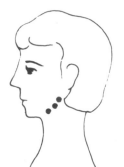

Fig. 89. Pressure on the carotid artery.

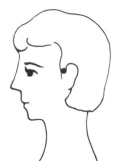

Fig. 90. Pressure on the lower jaw to the bottom of the ear.

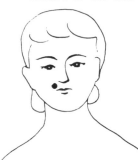

Fig. 91. Pressure on the area over the aching tooth.

Toothache

Toothaches, caused by decay, pyorrhea, gingivitis, periodontitis, and pulpitis demand the immediate attention of a dentist, but sometimes nervous tension can produce toothaches equally as painful as those arising from organic disorders. When this happens or when a patient, though under dental care, is nonetheless suffering, shiatsu treatment reduces and sometimes eliminates the pain completely.

1. Apply pressure to the carotid artery under the lower jaw on the same side as the aching tooth *(Fig. 89)*.

2. Press along the lower jaw to the lower part of the ear.

3. Apply strong pressure with three fingers to the temple. Repeat two or three times *(Fig. 90)*.

4. Using three fingers, apply pressure for an extended period on the portion of the cheek directly over the aching tooth *(Fig. 91)*. The pain will gradually subside.

Headache

Headaches often accompany toothaches, but whatever their cause, shiatsu is effective in treating them.

1. Have the patient lie on his back, and sit facing the top of his head.

2. Apply pressure to the key points of the median line from the hairline to the crown *(Fig. 92)*. Press all six points three times.

3. Press the three key points on the left and right of the crown four times.

4. Repeat step 2. Press each of the points on the side of the crown simultaneously six times.

5. Repeat step 2.

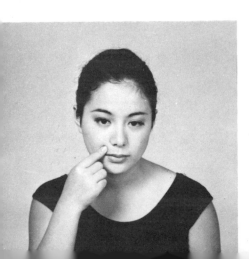

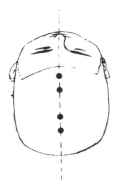

Fig. 92. The key points on the median line.

Rheumatism

Seldom responsive to medication, arthritic and rheumatic pains of the back and shoulder—called forties' back and fifties' shoulder in Japanese because they usually occur in people of those ages—respond readily to shiatsu treatment.

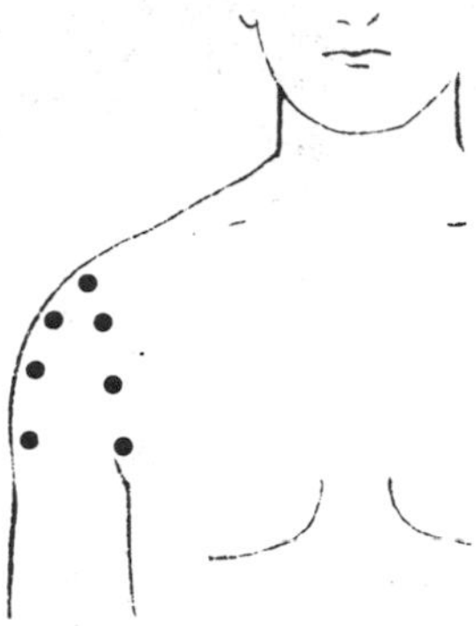

Rheumatic pains of the shoulders

1. Have the patient sit upright, and kneel beside him with one knee drawn up.
2. Apply pressure first to the three key points of the deltoid muscle in the shoulder, and then work downward *(Fig. 93)*. Repeat three times for two seconds each. When you reach the area of greatest pain, the patient will react, thus indicating the root of the trouble. Continued pressure on this point will ease the pain and relax the stiffness of the muscle.
3. Have the patient lie on his side with his back to you.
4. With one thumb on top of the other, apply pressure to the three points below the hollow of the scapula *(Fig. 94)*. Since this area will be very sensitive, begin with light pressure and gradually increase force.
5. A single treatment will enable the patient to raise the arms that formerly were in great pain, but twenty treatments will eradicate the difficulty completely. A hot bath after each treatment increases the effectiveness of the cure.

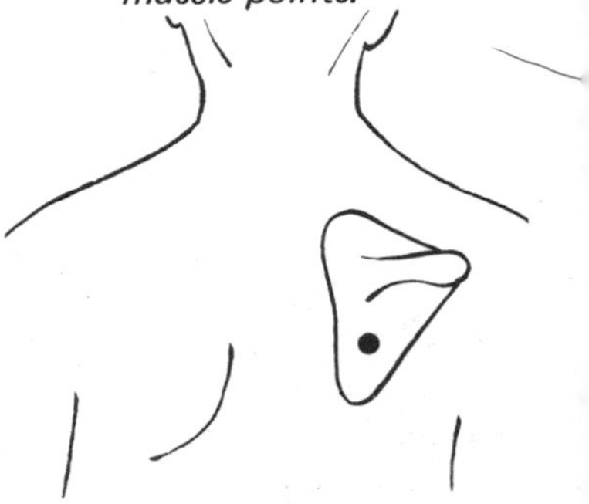

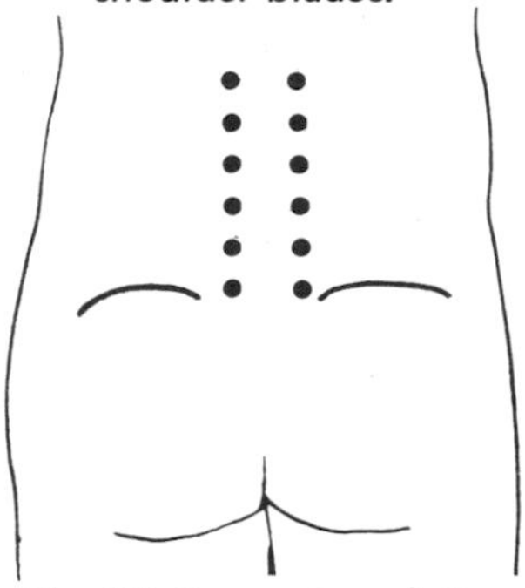

Rheumatic pains of the back

The following routine relieves the aching of the lumbar region common in middle-aged people who must sit or stand for long periods.

1. Have the patient lie facedown, and sit beside him.
2. Using three fingers, press the fifth lumbar vertebra lightly. The patient will feel pain at the spot requiring treatment.
3. First, apply pressure simultaneously with both thumbs to the muscles on either side of the vertebra, but not on the vertebra itself. After the surrounding muscles have relaxed, press the vertebra. Continue the pressure until the condition has been eased *(Fig. 95)*.
4. Have the patient lie on his back.
5. Sitting beside him, press lightly with the palm of the hand on the abdomen from the stomach to the colon. Press repeatedly on any hard area. When the abdomen is relaxed, the pains in the lumbar region will disappear *(Fig. 96)*.

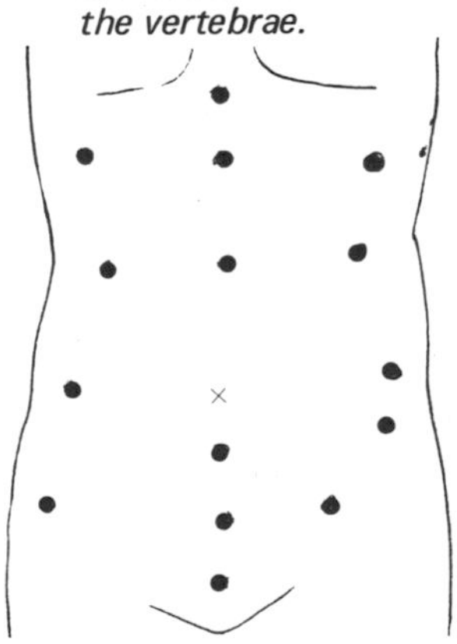

Fig. 93. The deltoid muscle points.

Fig. 94. Points below the hollow of the shoulder blades.

Fig. 95. Pressure points on either side of the vertebrae.

Fig. 96. The abdominal region.

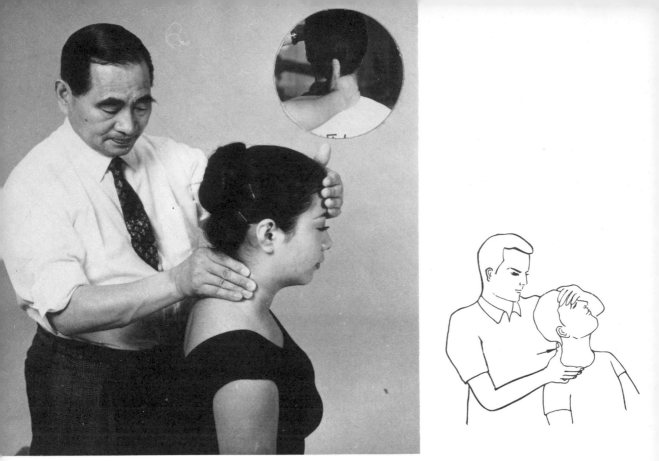

Fig. 97. Pressing the medulla oblongata to cure nosebleed.

Nosebleed

Nosebleed may occur in women six or seven months pregnant, or in anyone when climate, emotions, or nutrition change radically and suddenly. Attacks caused by sudden rushes of blood to the head and those in late stages of pregnancy, if accompanied by heavy head, bloodshot eyes, and flushed face, usually result from angioneurosis. Frequent bleeding from the nose should be treated by a doctor, but that caused by high blood pressure, compensatory menstruation, or emotional upset can be handled at home. If stanching is necessary, pack the nostrils with cotton wool or gauze, and if bleeding persists, chill the nasal region with a cold towel. The patient must lean his head back (*Fig. 97*).

1. Holding his forehead with your left hand, massage the points on the medulla oblongata with your right thumb till the bleeding stops.

Crick in the Neck

Cricks in the neck, caused by sleeping in an unnatural position, or in other parts of the body by sudden movement or attempts to lift something heavy cause excruciating pain and stiffness in all the surrounding muscles. Such surface symptoms, however, are only superficial manifestations of a deeper inability of the muscles to work together smoothly. Violent handling of the affected areas will only increase the pain and produce inflammation.

1. Treatment must reach the affected deep muscles, not just stiff surface ones. To locate the heart of the difficulty, press the aching part lightly. If pain is great, relax the area by warming it with the hand or a hot towel.

2. Apply shiatsu pressure as gently as if you were trying to coax your way by an armed sentry; force can do great damage.

3. Press gently until the surface disorder and, finally, the deeper trouble are cured. If the deep muscles are torn, recovery may take several days, but shiatsu should enable the patient to move the damaged part without extreme pain. Always treat stiffness in shoulders, the source of the more serious crick, at the first sign of discomfort.

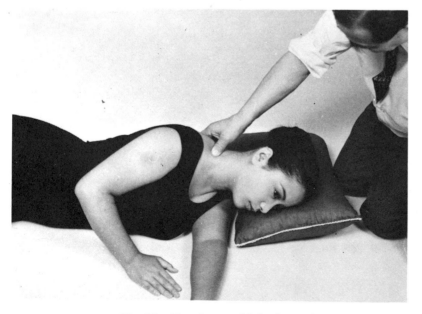

Fig. 98. Treating a crick in the neck.

Contusions and Sprains

Skiing and other sports provide good opportunities for healthful exercise, but they also take their yearly toll in bruises, fractures, contusions, and sprains. Although the external symptoms of a contusion may be so insignificant that the patient overlooks them, they develop impediments in the connective-tissue membranes and capillary blood vessels and thereby produce swelling, subcutaneous bleeding, and inflammation. Contusions demand immediate attention to prevent their after-affects lingering to become serious.

Sprains, caused by forcible action on a joint or irregular movement exceeding the joint's normal capacity, result in damage to the joint capsule and ligament and cause such pain that practically no one ever ignores them. Though they stop just short of the dislocation stage, they are sometimes extremely troublesome, and take a long time to cure.

1. Use palm pressure on the affected area with one hand because both contusions and sprains produce swelling and sometimes sharp pain.

2. Press lightly on the damaged part until the feverishness and throbbing subside.

3. Beginning at the upper zone of the damage, execute the proper shiatsu treatment on the injured member.

4. Apply shiatsu pressure thoroughly to the muscles connected with the injured part. This treatment should accelerate recovery.

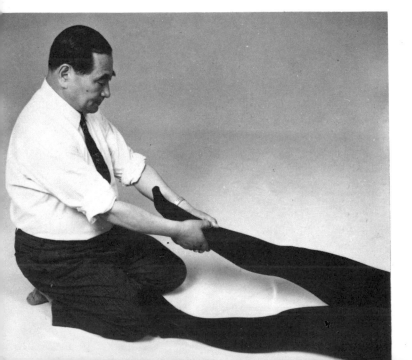

Fig. 99. Treating an injured leg.

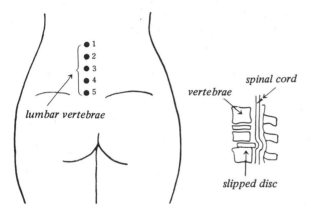

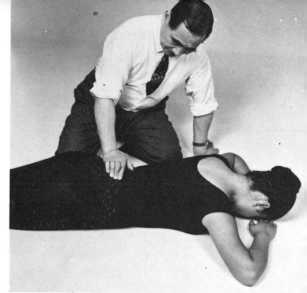

Fig. 100. Treatment of a slipped spinal disc.

Slipped Spinal Disc

Dislocations of the discs located among vertebrae and consequent pressure on the spinal cord, a common complaint today, are usually caused by falls, lifting something heavy, or twisting the waist suddenly and unnaturally. Treat such cases in the following way.

1. Ask the patient where the pain is. It is usually the fourth or fifth lumbar vertebra, but you must discern whether the right or left side of the vertebra is involved *(Fig. 100)*.

2. (I will assume that the problem concerns the left side of the fourth lumbar vertebra.) Avoiding abrupt pressure, relieve the stiffness of the muscle on the left side of that vertebra by continual pressure with the thumbs.

3. Next, using the bulb of the middle finger, softly press the concave spot between the spinous processes of the fourth and fifth lumbar vertebrae. The acute pain the patient feels reveals this as the source of the trouble. Press lightly for a duration of one second; repeat five times.

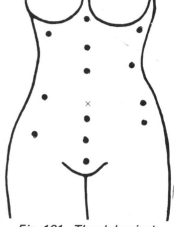

Fig. 101. The abdominal region.

4. Have the patient turn over on his back, and apply shiatsu pressure with the fingers and the palm to his abdominal region. Pay particularly close attention to the pit of the stomach *(Fig. 101)*.

5. Press the left side of the navel gently but deeply.

6. The patient will complain of pain somewhere near the lumbar region; apply palm pressure to that point ten times for about three seconds each.

7. The patient should lie still for a while and avoid bending and twisting for the next few days.

Cholelithiasis (Gallstone Colic)

Cholesterol and other substances transformed into calculi, or stones, in the gall bladder cause the pain felt in various parts of the body (right shoulder, right scapula, third, fourth, fifth, and sixth interscapular points) in cases of cholelithiasis. The following treatment is effective.

1. Have the patient lie on his right side.
2. Apply shiatsu pressure thoroughly and repeatedly to the entire region, beginning at the upper part of the right shoulder and including the right scapula and the interscapular region down to the lumbar region *(Fig. 102)*.
3. Next, have the patient turn over on his back, and press repeatedly on the upper part of the right side of the abdomen *(Fig. 103)*.

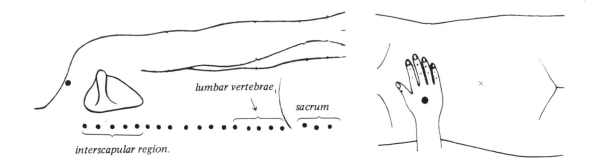

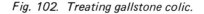

Fig. 102. *Treating gallstone colic.*   Fig. 103. *Pressure on the abdomen.*

Bedwetting

Incontinence of the urine stems from a dulled reaction in the sphincter of the bladder. Excess intake of liquids and chill during sleep also bring on bedwetting in people who are likely to have stiff lumbar and abdominal muscles. Treat as follows.

1. Press the five points on both sides of the lumbar region and then the three points in the sacrum *(Fig. 104)*.
2. Next, with the palm of the hand, press the lower abdomen, particularly the area over the bladder *(Fig. 106)*.
3. Finally, apply pressure to the medulla oblongata *(Fig. 105)*.

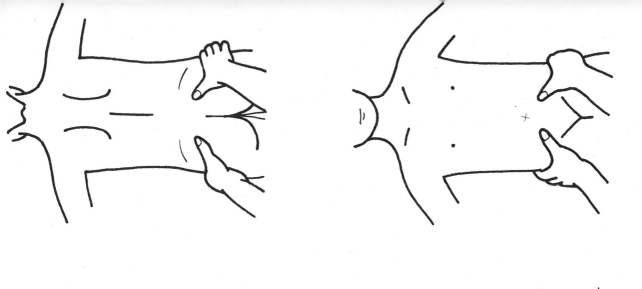

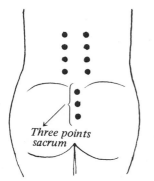

Fig. 104. Points on either side of
the lumbar vertebrae and
on the sacrum.

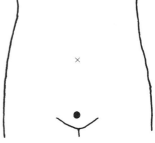

Fig. 105. Medulla oblongata.

Fig. 106. Lower abdomen.

Infant Care

Shiatsu as a regular part of baby care, performed during the diaper change or the bath, by increasing the infant's appetite and promoting healthy bowel action contributes to fast growth.

1. First, lightly place the palm of your hand on the baby's navel for about ten seconds; then increase the pressure slightly. Repeat this pressure five times, two seconds each (Fig. 106).

2. Next, press lightly on the pit of the stomach with the bulbs of the index finger, middle finger, and fourth finger. Using very light pressure, repeat three times, two seconds each.

3. Next, press lightly on the area below the navel and over the bladder. Using three fingers, press three times.

4. Finally, with the palm of the hand press five times on the navel.

Wryneck

Infantile wryneck may be congenital, or it may be caused by careless parents who allow the baby to sleep predominantly on one side. Started early, shiatsu treatment can cure the shrinkage of the sternomastoid muscle (extending from behind the ear lobe to the tip of the clavicle) that causes this unfortunate condition *(Fig. 100)*.

1. Using the thumb and working downward apply shiatsu pressure to the hardened muscle you will find at the side of the baby's contracted neck.

2. Next, press the three points in the front of the neck from below the ear to the tip of the shoulder; repeat ten times.

3. Press the three points on the side of the neck ten times.

Repeat this series of pressure applications three times daily, but be very gentle. Since the neck is flexible, cure is possible if treatment is thorough and persistent.

Fig. 107. Curing wryneck.

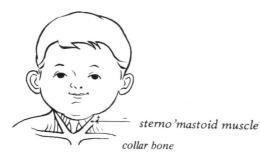

sterno'mastoid muscle

collar bone

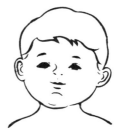

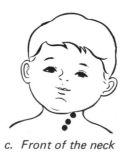

a. *Back of the neck.*　　　b. *Side of the neck.*　　　c. *Front of the neck*

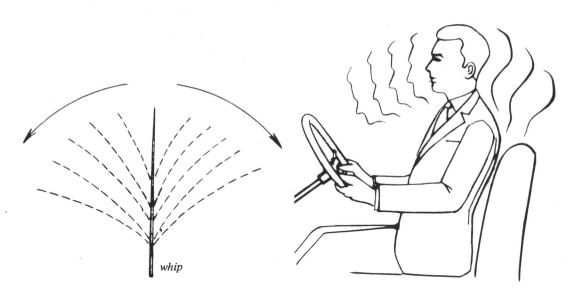

Fig. 108. The action of a whip and the similar movement caused in the human body by sudden braking of an automobile.

Whiplash Injuries

The contemporary traffic war has created a new kind of injury: displacement of the seven cervical vertebrae in the neck as the result of violent shakes administered to the trunk of the body in sudden braking and automobile crashes. Resulting compression of the nerves in the neck*(Fig. 109)*produces headaches, dizziness, pains in the neck, and numb arms that sometimes last for a long times and disrupt work and social life. When the shock of a crash results in loss of consciousness, call a physician immediately. For persistent aftereffects of whiplash, follow this routine.
1. Press the side and back of the neck, and the area from the medulla oblongata to the base of the neck. This should return the muscles of the neck, consequently, the slipped bones to their normal positions.
2. Sometimes X-rays will not reveal distortions that cause painful symptoms; therefore, in any injury involving a suspicion of the whiplash effect, an immediate application of shiatsu pressure is a good idea.

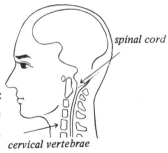

spinal cord

cervical vertebrae

Fig. 109. Treating the whiplash effect.

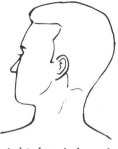

twisted cervical muscles

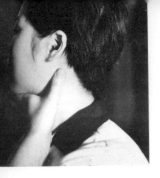

Motion Sickness

When car sickness is autosuggestive and results from a neurosis or weak digestion, first press the mastoid process (bone protruding behind the ear *(Fig. 111)*., then the medulla oblongata, nape of the neck, shoulders, and interscapular area. As stiffness in that area disappears, so will the car sickness.

It is also important to remember that car sickness sometimes arises from a sensitivity to the smell of gasoline. In such cases, provide plenty of fresh air. If sudden stopping, turning, high speeds, or bad roads seem to cause the trouble, have the person affected get out of the car for a moment and apply strong pressure to the mastoid process and the pit of the stomach.

Sickness from riding on trains is caused by insufficient food or sleep, or from sitting too long with the result that blood does not circulate to the head properly and the limbs become very tired.

To bring quick relief, press the sanri points *(Fig. 110)* in the legs, the plantar arches, the medulla oblongata, and the nape of the neck.

Sickness on aircraft, largely psychological, is best relieved by conversing with someone or reading something light. The discomfort caused in the ears by pressure change will vanish if you chew gum, eat a little candy, talk, or do anything that keeps the mouth moving so that the pressure differential between the cabin and the inside of the head can equalize quickly. Shiatsu pressure on the mastoid process, the temples, medulla oblongata, and the nape of the neck is effective.

When seasick, remain quiet, and apply pressure to the mastoid process, the abdomen (especially the gastric region), the upper shoulder, and the backbone. This will promote appetite so that the patient can eat lightly.

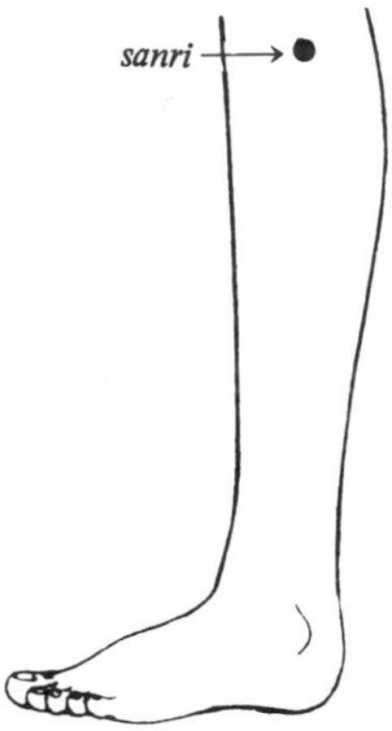

sanri →

Fig. 110. Pressure on the sanri helps stimulate circulation and thereby dispel motion sickness caused by long train rides.

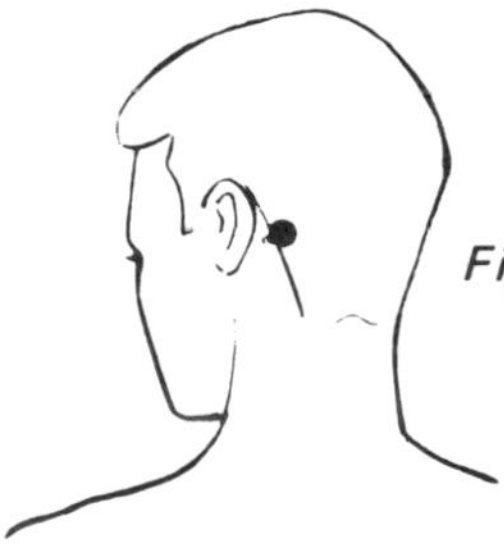

Fig. 111. To relieve motion sickness, press the mastoid process.

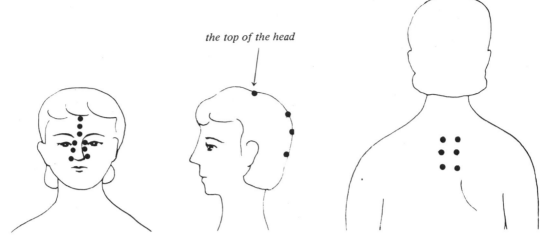

the top of the head

Fig. 112. *Pressure to relieve sinusitis.*   Fig. 113. *Pressure to relieve asthma discomforts.*

Sinusitis

Pus accumulating in the course of infection in the paranasal sinuses (ducts connecting the frontal and maxillary sinuses) produces the condition known as sinusitis in which the nose discharges a green fluid and is congested, the head aches, causing negative thinking and bad memory.

For relief, press both sides of the nose and the forehead, the parietal bone, the front, side, and back of the neck, the medulla oblongata, and the upper shoulders *(Fig.112)*.

Asthma

To relieve the coughing and congestion of asthmatic attacks, press the right and left sides of the body (particularly the interscapular region), the back of the neck (three point on each side, *Fig. 113)*, and the thoracic vertebrae.
1. During the attack, have the patient lie on his back without a pillow, and with four fingers on the back of his neck, press points three and four on the front of the neck with your thumb.
2. Put a pillow under his head, and apply pressure to his chest with a circular motion of the palms of both hands. Repeat ten times; then press straight down on the chest twice to promote exhalation. Finally press his abdomen.

Writer's Cramp

Chronic fatigue in the muscles of the forearms produces this form of dyskinesia, common among writers and painters.

1. Press the points of the front, side, and back of the neck, the upper shoulders, and the infraspinous fossa (hollow of the scapula).
2. Give the arms, particularly the forearms and the *sanri*, wrists, hands, and fingers a thorough shiatsu treatment.
3. Press the back of the hand (between the metacarpal bones) at three points on each space beginning near the thumb, above and below the fingers, and on both sides of each finger. Finally press the three points on the palm of the hand.

Cramps of the Calf (Gastrocnemius Muscle)

Cramps of the large muscle of the calf result from fatigue and disturbances of the internal organs, chilled limbs or lumbar region, or trouble in the sciatic nerve.

1. Apply strong pressure to the trochanter major.
2. Press the three points on the back of the thigh and on the back of the knee.
3. Press the eight points on the leg leading to the ankle *(Fig.114)*.
4. Press the *sanri* points, then the knee, ankle, and sole.

Frequent shiatsu applied to the entire body, particularly the lower half, helps prevent these cramps.

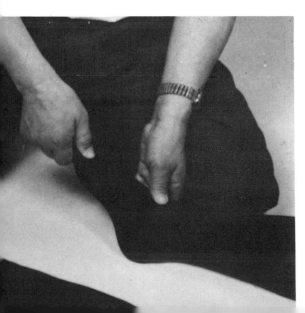

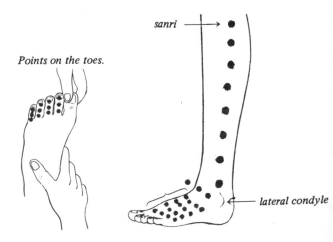

Points on the toes.

sanri

lateral condyle

Fig. 114. Points on leg and foot.

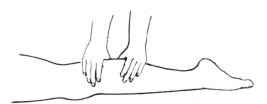

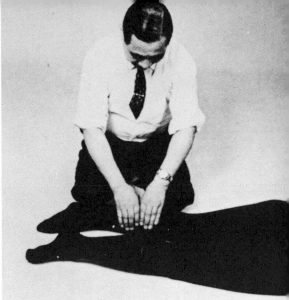

Fig. 115. Numbness of the leg.

Numbness in the Legs

When kneeling or sitting for a long time has numbed your legs, stretch them out, apply strong shiatsu pressure to the eight points on the calf, massage the six points of the ankle with both hands, press the sanri point, and then the ankle and sole (*Fig. 115*).

Index